VICTORY OVER ARTHRITIS

by Rasmus Alsaker, M.D.

1966 Edition by

GROTON PRESS, INC.

74 THIRD AVENUE   BROOKLYN, NEW YORK

CONTENTS

III FOODS AND COOKING

I CAUSATION OF ARTHRITIS AND RHEUMATISM

1 Greetings

More than forty years of work, study and experience have gone into this book, although the recording has taken only a few months. Friends have repeatedly asked for a treatise on arthritis and rheumatism that could be used as a home guide. One friend and former patient from Florida has requested that each chapter be headed with a letter from a recovered patient; also that a history of my work in this field should serve as an introduction. He is very enthusiastic about this record and has endorsed the work extensively; here is a part of one of his statements: "My arthritis of back, shoulders and legs cleared up, after it had been impressed on me by others that this could not be done." He was instructed in healthful ways of living, so he could remain well afterwards, if he so desired.

We are unable to comply with the request of

beginning each chapter with a letter from a recovered patient, for a doctor is so trained into thinking that the physician-patient relationship is
personal and privileged and confidential that he
is unable to ask such permission from his patients.
But stories will be told about patients, taking good
care that they cannot be identified.

As for the history of our work in this field, you
may find it helpful in making your decisions, so
we shall give it briefly:

CURABILITY OF ARTHRITIS

When we attended medical college over forty
years ago we were informed that arthritis is incurable. The professor of the Practice of Medicine told
us that we would have to treat these patients even
if we could not help them. Various salicylates were
recommended, for they relieve pain without causing drug addiction. Aside from drugging, no important recommendations were given except the standard, "make the patient comfortable," and "give him
plenty of good nourishing food," both of which
were repeated at nearly every lecture.

Why was arthritis looked upon as incurable? Because there was such a firm faith in drugs that no
other treatment was attempted among the majority of physicians.

We knew before attending medical school that

arthritis was curable, for we had seen several men and women recover by changing their way of eating and drinking, and being more careful to obtain a good bowel movement every day. To those who have not given this matter thought, this may seem odd, even impossible. But please let us tell you the facts:

A great building is as good as the materials put into it, and the skill of the architect and the workmen. By using good steel, building blocks, mortar, cement, and other materials of high quality, plus a fine foundation and roof, with good workmanship you get a sound building.

The human structure is built of food, water and air. If these three are skillfully combined, and the body is kept clean, a sound physical structure is the result, provided it is kept internally clean. Being highly intelligent, the human body is greatly affected by the mental state; depressive thinking and emotionalism tend to diminish health, while uplifting or constructive thinking and emotionalism help to rebuild and maintain health.

And so it is that food, water, air and internal cleanliness may be employed to overcome arthritis; constructive, courageous thinking is a great help. An uplifted mind aids in toning up the body.

Although we do not have the records of our first year of practice, memory says that among the patients there were many arthritics. We had no years of starving, but enjoyed a good practice from the start. Nearly all of the arthritics made satisfactory recoveries. A few came after the affected joints had greatly deteriorated, and these joints did not become as good as new, although nearly all of them improved and lost their pain, discomfort and some of their immobility. Those who had no serious joint deterioration did well and made as full recovery as they desired. Not all will be careful enough to return to the best health possible.

This answers the most-asked question in and about arthritis: "Can one recover from arthritis?" We shall restate the answer in one sentence: Yes, if arthritis is taken in reasonable time, recovery is the rule, but if the condition is permitted to continue till the joints are wrecked, the joints cannot be fully restored, although considerable mobility may be regained and usually the pain and discomfort vanish. Fortunately, most of the arthritics are seen in time for a fine recovery.

As the years went on so many arthritics came to us that many thought we specialized in this disease, which we did not. We now wish we had kept a permanent record of them, but we are sure that we have had such patients by the thousands. The results have been most satisfying. Of course, we have had many who did not continue until the results were complete, many who would not work with us until they had gathered all the knowledge of correct living needed to stay well.

Arthritis, which is inflammation of the joints,

may occur at any age, but it is most common in the forties and the fifties; once established, it generally remains for life, unless one learns how to live so as to overcome it. Please let me repeat an oft-told tale, one of the most dramatic in the annals of my practice because of the age of one of the patients.

STORIES FROM LIFE

A homemaker came to us with this story: "I love to dance, but my knees won't let me. I did not mind the arthritis so much when it affected my hands and arms; it was not very painful, but now it is limiting my motions; it is hard to go down steps and stairs and I have to pay a high price for just one waltz. What can you do for me?" She was about fifty years of age, had a good family history, seemed to possess a good constitution, and had no other diseases. She had been healthy until the previous year.

So we explained that with the best of care and cooperation she should improve enough so she could begin dancing again within four months, possibly in three months. She was a splendid patient, and lost all swelling, soreness and pain in less than two months; in about three months she was dancing in moderation; she gradually increased the time on the dance floor until she could dance as much as the rest of her social set.

Not along after her recovery she consulted us about her mother: "I suppose nothing can be done for Mother; she has arthritis, but she is seventy-eight years of age; I want to be sure." She said her mother was cheery and hopeful—how different from most arthritics! She came from healthy stock, with many old people in the family.

So we informed her that recovery had only a little to do with age; it depends mostly on the patient's vitality, constitution and state of mind. The idea that a person past seventy cannot he helped is not true, if these factors are favorable. It may take a little longer to recover, for there is a general rule that the older one is, the slower the recovery.

So the mother, who had been a prisoner in her own home for some months, was brought to the daughter's home where we met her. She was a delightful young woman of seventy-eight, keen of mind and interested in the affairs of the world; arthritis was her only ill, so it was safe to give the verdict that she could make a good recovery. She did, at the same time losing her excessive weight. Six months later we had a letter from a young relative in Boston that this "incurable" patient had spent a whole Saturday shopping, wearing out her young companions. We heard from her occasionally for the next thirteen years; we were informed by another relative when she was ninety-one years of age that she was keen of mind, spry and active of body and that she was enjoying life.

She was fortunate in having a fine, vital husmand. Although he was four years older than his wife he was sharing his wife's physical and mental activities. When we first met him he could no longer preach because of clergyman's sore throat, which is a mixture of laryngitis and chronic catarrh. He was instructed in a few changes to make in his eating and living habits. Would you believe it? He happily returned to his preaching! This man and wife were truly young in mind and spirit, although elderly as we measure time for human beings. They were among the most delightful patients we have known.

For about four years we were the professional head of a sanitarium, where we relied on sunlight, good air, plenty of water, good natural food, internal cleanliness, and far from least, a hopeful constructive psychology. The results were gratifying. As no one else was grounded in the psychology of health, we had to furnish that in weekly lectures and consultations with the patients. To show you what beneficial effects the right psychology has on the sick, when we left, the patients became upset and unhappy—no, no, not because of our leaving, but because there was no one to furnish them with the right psychology, the mental uplift that is so important in building health.

It was in this institution we met our Florida friend and helped him to break the bonds of arthritis. Some odd reactions occurred there. Ar-

thritis is a difficult disease that reluctantly permits
a patient to escape, but, after a stay of three days
with us, one arthritic complained, "Doctor, I still
have arthritis." It is astonishing how many arthritics look for miracles—and occasionally one
seems to occur: For instance, a woman of sixty-
two had such severe arthritis that she could no
longer attend morning mass, nor could she lift her
arms high enough to arrange her hair. She carefully followed instructions for three days, and resumed full physical activity, including daily morning mass. It seems impossible, but it happened—
we make no attempt to explain it. We knew her
for some years thereafter; every time we saw her
son, which was frequently, he said, "Mother is doing fine in every way."

The facts about the results we obtained spread
near and far. An eminent physician came to visit
and investigate us. We gave him full freedom to
watch and investigate; he was permitted to read
charts; to visit with the patients and get their stories and ask them about the results; to inspect our
physical therapy department and talk with our
technicians—we gave him carte blanche. He saw
what we did and talked with many patients about
the results, and they told us that he went around
muttering, "It can't be so," "such results are impossible," and similar phrases; finally he rushed out of
our institution without one word of thanks for the
courtesies we had extended to him. Of course, it

is understandable that seeing so many things happening that he had looked upon as impossible, in such a short time, would disturb him. He saw what we did not only for arthritis and rheumatism, but for chronic bronchitis, asthma, ulcers, nephritis and many other difficult diseases.

Our Florida friend, who was a pharmacist, also saw these things and was impressed so much that he still is enthusiastic about Nature's Way of dealing with disease. It is too bad that this sanitarium is no longer in existence.

But let us return to the woman who had such speedy results. In three days she lost her soreness, stiffness, pain and disability; but she did not recover in that short time; she was still very toxic, so we supervised her until she overcame the toxicity, until we had time to train her into right eating and right living in general so she would remain well, if she lived up to Nature's Way of overcoming and preventing arthritis.

After leaving the sanitarium we resumed private practice in New York City. Most of the patients have been and still are the victims of chronic disease—many of these can be classed as diseases of chronic degeneration. Arthritics and rheumatics have been prominent among them. Many have made good recoveries; some have quit as soon as they improved enough to be comfortable, without obtaining the knowledge necessary for future health, which is always an unhappy termination. It is so satisfying to do a good job.

A few months ago a grandmother from a Rocky Mountain state was speculating that her active days were a thing of the past, for she was over seventy and suffering with arthritis. But she decided to give us and Nature's Way a chance. She was an excellent patient and in less than three months she was able to go fishing with her grandchildren, which thrilled and delighted them.

But not all get such quick results. One woman, over fifty years of age, had no stride four months ago, more than a decade of arthritis having reduced her to pitiful mincing steps. What a pleasure it is to see her stride forth now; it is wonderful to regain one's stride after it has been lost. Her recovery is slow, but steady; she looks so much better and she is growing stronger in hope and faith.

"Do you truly want to recover?" we often ask our seriously ill patients who talk or act in an irresponsible way. And that is no joke, for recovering from serious disease takes earnestness and character; it requires tenacity of purpose. But the rewards are so great! The real price of recovery is right living; this has been known to a few for a long time —we have attempted to broadcast this truth in all directions.

The good news is that arthritis taken in reasonable time can be overcome by natural methods; if the patient lets the disease continue until the joints are badly injured, full recovery is often out of the question, but improvement can generally take place.

2 What Causes Arthritis

This is an important question because we must know much about the causation before we can give the correct treatment. And it is especially important when we realize that perhaps eight millions of the population of these United States suffer with chronic rheumatic or arthritic ills; furthermore, that arthritis cripples more human beings than any other disease.

Rheumatism and arthritis go together in the minds of doctors; the definition and separation of these two ills are not always sharp.

But technically, arthritis is inflammation of the joints, usually with swelling, and often with degeneration. Not only the joints, but the surrounding structures are usually involved. If the inflammation is bad, the articulating surfaces deteriorate and roughen; the tough membranes covering the bones (the periosteum), the ligaments and the smooth membrane (synovial membrane) of the joints, the special cartilages covering the joint surfaces, and the bones surrounding the joints are affected. The bones lose some of their calcium, and the joints swell. This is arthritis.

The joints are lubricated with an albuminous fluid derived from the blood plasma—not with oil. Unfortunately, those who lack both knowledge and experience write for arthritics; we have before us literature showing how the best means of ridding the body of arthritis is to get plenty of oil into the joints; and the way is described of eating oil so that it will escape digestion and thus be absorbed and carried to the joints for lubricating purposes. But things do not happen that way in the body—the blood does not carry globules of fat and deposit them in the joints, and, we repeat, oil is not the lubricating fluid of the joints.

Rheumatism is a flexible term indicating painful states that may originate in muscles, nerves, tendons, joints and even bones. When we diagnose carefully, we generally come to more definite terms, such as neuritis, and bursitis. On the whole, we find it best to call inflammation of the joints arthritis, and reserve rheumatism for inflammatory states of softer tissues, with pain.

But what causes this disease, which disables more human beings than all accidents that occur, and far more than any other disease? We shall deal in this discussion chiefly with the four forms of arthritis (according to the American Rheumatism

Association) that make up about 95% of all
arthritis:

1 RHEUMATOID ARTHRITIS
   of the peripheral joints
   of the spine, or spondylitis
2 DEGENERATIVE JOINT DISEASE
   localized
   generalized
3 FIBROSITIS
   localized
   generalized
4 ARTHRITIS DUE TO GOUT

And it is well to note here that the other forms
of arthritis (5% or less) are attributed to bacteria,
other diseases, injury or wounds, nervous conditions, neoplasms or tumors, hydrarthrosis, drugs,
serums and even hysteria. There is no complete
agreement on this subject, but this gives a very
good idea what the conventional views are.

As for the causation, it is rather well agreed
among physicians that no specific cause is known,
and that no special treatment is indicated.

But we feel certain we know the cause, that we
have known it for decades, for based on our own
formulated causation we have helped thousands
of arthritic victims to recover, and we have given
them the knowledge to keep them well. This is so
important in dealing with this tyrannical disease

that we hope you will give full attention to the rest of this chapter.

AUTOINTOXICATION

It is natural to be healthy. Babies, born of healthy parents, come into life normal, if there are no accidents. This is the general rule. With the right care in infancy and childhood, the baby grows and develops into a healthy adult.

Men and women can remain healthy during the middle years—they do not have to deteriorate. By living right they maintain themselves in good condition until they are sixty, seventy and older. Good health is the normal state; disease is abnormal. But we need the correct living knowledge, and the stamina, will power practiced, to put it into our living. This is a low price to pay for health.

However, fine health during the middle years is the exception. Some are in tolerable health, but the majority entertain limiting diseases; half of the population develops diseases of the heart and arteries; millions cultivate arthritis. So it is that when they should be at their best, multitudes live so as to be uncomfortable, weakened, distressed and unhappy; men lose their strength; women, their beauty, for disease, not age, is the greatest destroyer of beauty of face and figure. Health, with inner poise, is the supreme beautifier.

Why are so many ill? Because they do not follow Nature's Way in their living mode, and consequently they become toxic. Right living prevents the autointoxication.

Normal babies start with a constitution and vitality to live more than one hundred years, if the living care is correct. But despite this, numerous talented human beings die before they can do and give their best. The reason is they do not realize that human life is built on law and order, and we have to obey the law if we desire health.

So long as we have health, we take it for granted. This is a mistake, for our civilization is so complex and unnatural that we must take special precautions to remain well. Civilization coops many of us up in cities where living quarters are too crowded, the air contaminated. So we exercise and breathe too little; we pamper the skin with excessive covering while living in too warm rooms; the digestion and elimination deteriorate—all of which tends towards increasing toxicity, or autointoxication.

AUTOINTOXICATION CAUSES DISEASE

What is autointoxication? It is a condition in which the body is poisoned throughout by its own excretions, because they are permitted to accumulate in the body before being expelled. These waste products, many of them the acids of oxidation, should be eliminated promptly; when they are not, they cause autointoxication. Some of these wastes are of bacterial origin, but most of them are debris that results from the slow combustion always taking place in the body, much of it in the muscles. This process is essential to life and produces heat and water and waste—the ashes of the fires of life within our bodies. Sluggish elimination from the four great eliminating organs—not from the bowels alone—results in the toxic state, or autointoxication. This should not be, but it happens to most human beings.

It is this evil, unclean condition within the body that is the basic cause of arthritis.

At first there are no bad symptoms of autointoxication. Later the results are too frequently serious. Here are some of the signs and symptoms that show up in time: A coated tongue, usually worst in the morning; bad breath, frequent colds, skin eruptions—all of these show lack of internal cleanliness. The skin often becomes muddy and coarse; the eye balls lose their lustre; the hair lacks tone; and irritability and nervousness are common symptoms.

Fugitive pains indicate autointoxication—cleanse the body and the pains vanish. But if the toxic condition is permitted to exist, rheumatism, arthritis and other ills often appear on the scene.

A healthy person arises refreshed and happy in the morning, but a toxic one needs coffee or some other bracer to come to full life. The normal thing is to be keen and bright in the morning, without stimulation.

If the early signs are heeded and the living habits are changed so the body is cleansed throughout, no harm is done. But let the toxicity persist and first comes acute disease, and after a while the chronic form.

Disease is the protest of the body against abuse.

Disease is an effort to throw off accumulated toxic waste—all waste created by a body is poisonous to that body. The body becomes feverish because it has to burn up the accumulated trash. If the body is permitted to burn up the acid wastes, and the living is changed for the better, health is the result; but if the toxic condition continues, various diseases may result, prominent among them rheumatism and arthritis.

Chronic diseases, arthritis included, can be prevented by giving the body correct care, but human beings are careless and most of them like to live as they were raised, so far as food is concerned.

It is natural to be well; it is abnormal to be toxic, so let us explain

HOW AUTOINTOXICATION DEVELOPS

1 The most obvious factor is wrong eating. The majority eat wrong from childhood; they develop bad habits that cling throughout life. The food we

need nourishes us; all we eat above our needs makes us sick. Overeating is a common cause of autointoxication and disease. Most families eat freely of cereals, bread, butter, meat, white sugar and rich desserts like cake, pie, pudding and cookies, and this kind of eating tends towards toxicity and disease. The majority undereat of fresh fruits and vegetables, which are on the side of health; they are the alkalizers and accordingly counteract overacidity, which is a toxic factor. Milk is also an alkalizer, but it is plentifully consumed, especially in childhood.

White sugar and white flour and their products are especially destructive of health—yes, even the enriched white flour. They are lacking in mineral salts and vitamins, factors essential to health. The body has to be mildly alkaline or neutral to be well, but the majority of adults suffer with too low alkalinity, which easily runs into autointoxication and disease, and much of that disease turns out to be rheumatism and arthritis.

2 Lack of internal cleanliness is the second cause of the toxic state, followed by arthritis. Internal cleanliness drives arthritis away. The four chief organs of elimination or internal cleansing are:

The lungs, which carry away the carbon dioxide or carbonic acid gas, and supply refreshing oxygen to the body; oxygen supports internal combustion, which is the fire of life that normally continues from the formation of the body in the womb to death.

However, the majority exercise and breathe too little to support this function in full, and many inhale bad air.

The skin is the second great cleansing system. It contains millions of pores through which acids and other wastes escape in a watery solution. If a large area of skin is destroyed, high fever ensues; if a very large area is destroyed, life ends, because the skin is so necessary to protect the underlying tissues, and to carry out of the body various toxic matters. The skin is overprotected and hence too sluggish to do its work fully. This means a slow gathering of impurities within the body.

The kidneys are the third set of cleansing organs, so important because they help to eliminate the most poisonous by-products of systemic activity, such as urates and uric acid, which come from the burning of proteins within the body. They need plenty of water to do their work well, otherwise some of the wastes of protein combustion are retained, and these are the most poisonous of all wastes. Many drink only one or two glasses of water a day, saying they take fruit juices, soup, milk, coffee and tea; but that will not do, for the juices, soups and milk are foods; coffee and tea are truly drugs, containing the poison caffeine. All should drink enough water, and those who fail to do so store up toxic waste or autointoxication, after which there is a strong tendency for the system to build chronic disease, arthritis included. A small woman needs at least five glasses of water per day; a larger one and men should have six or more glasses of water daily to keep the body sweet and clean and free from toxic compounds. Underdrinking of water is one of the chief causes of arthritis. Water is the best cleanser we have; this is as true of the inner body as it is of the body surface and the clothes we wear.

The fourth cleansing organ is the large intestine or colon, which eliminates the coarse waste from the body. It must be kept clean at all times, for if it is not, much of the toxic matter is reabsorbed, to be circulated once more through the blood and the lymph to cause the toxic state, and to help to produce headaches, pimples, rheumatism, arthritis, bronchitis and many other evils, known as disease. Constipation is a national curse. How sad it is that so many do not know that constipation poisons the body, which builds up autointoxication, which in turn produces disease, rheumatism and arthritis included! Many do not realize that the bowels should act fully every day! Even some physicians, who should know the vital facts, advise that it is all right to go two or even three days without a good bowel action! Some take cathartics and say they are normal. Then, why do they take the cathartics? A normal person needs no remedies for the bowels. Nine out of ten adults over forty are more or less constipated. Lack of a sweet, clean colon is one of the outstanding causes of rheumatism and arthritis. Please remember that autointoxication means self-poisoning, that one way of building this self-poisoning is constipation, and furthermore that this self-poisoning or autointoxication is the basic cause of rheumatism and arthritis.

A dirty face causes no physical harm, but a dirty bowel can and often does mean tragedy after the age of forty or fifty years.

Perhaps we should have placed subnormal water drinking in a class by itself as a cause of arthritis and rheumatism, for it always results in autointoxication, and is an outstanding cause of rheumatism and arthritis. So we repeat on purpose:

A small person should drink at least five glasses of water each day; a large person should drink more.

3 The third great cause of rheumatism and arthritis is mental-emotional. This is a little difficult to explain because it is intangible. But the truth is that the mind is the leader and the guide of the body. The unconscious mind, a part of the mind we are unable to use in our reasoning processes, commands, yes, commands the heart, the lungs, the kidneys, the liver and the digestive processes. Yes, the unconscious mind takes care of our vital organs so as to keep us alive. The emotions are another part of the mind that we may direct so as to help us build health or produce disease, depending on the kind of emotional life we choose.

Wrong thinking is the negative, depressing, destructive way of directing the thoughts and emotions. If we could get this basic truth to all readers, it would be a tremendous service to humanity. But thoughts are intangible, so these facts are difficult for many to grasp, and evaluate. Worry, fear, discouragement, apprehension, anxiety, depression and related emotions not only pull down the body and mind, but a little known scientific truth is that all of the depressing thoughts and emotions create poisons within the body, slow down and even stop some of the physical functions, such as digestion, and thus create disease; or they may speed up an organ abnormally, such as the effect of anger on the heart. Another effect of the destructive emotions is constriction, or contraction or tension of parts of the body, often through the neck and shoulders. When not in use the body should be relaxed and easy, ever ready to do its work.

When tensions are bad, people say they are nervous, and as the nerves are at fault they can't do anything about it. This is a mistake; it is not the nerves, but the mind that is in turmoil; calm down the mind, including the emotions, and the nervousness grows less and less. To function in health, the mind must be at peace and ease most of the time. No one expects perfection in this direction, but inner peace a large part of the time is one part of the price we have to pay for good health.

In the past forty years we have seen four patients killed by intense fear, shock and anger, caused by the folly of family or outsiders. For instance, a member of her congregation scared a young mother, who clasped her delicate boy to her breast; he nursed, and died in convulsions a few hours later, poisoned by his mother's milk.

Briefly, the causes of rheumatism and arthritis are partly physical mistakes, partly mental-emotional errors. We have confidence in this statement because it has been our privilege to see thousands of arthritics lose their soreness, stiffness, aches and pains by replacing the wrong ways of life with correct living modes.

Please consider the fact that we have long known that our domestic animals thrive when correctly fed and kindly treated. We human beings also are beings of flesh and blood. The same natural law applies to us: Living according to the laws of Nature, physical and mental, that rule our lives, and we fare well; but go contrary to those laws, and we fare ill.

So we shall show you how to avoid the by-paths of life that lead to disease, and travel the broad highway of health.

3 The Emotions and Arthritis

One of the greatest causes of arthritis is depressive emotionalism. It is difficult to explain, but there is no doubt about the facts. Such powerful emotions as anger and hatred, when fully unleashed, stop some of the physical functions and pervert them. Most of those much given to bad temper can remember how a fit of anger produced indigestion. This emotion is so powerful that it can even kill a human being. Years ago a young woman with serious leakage of the heart consulted us. We told her that if she would calm down she could lead a pleasant life, but that she had to discontinue all strenuous physical activities and emotional sprees—she lacked self-discipline.

For a few months she was a good patient in every way; her improvement astonished patient and family alike. When she came to the point that she could say, "I feel fine every day," she decided to go to a neighboring city and make a series of visits. We explained to her that her good feelings were not only due to good behavior, but dependent on it; that if she became careless about food and drink, and exhausted herself at all-night parties, her heart would surely cause trouble again within a few weeks. For three weeks she had a hilarious time, no limitations, no self-discipline. And then she collapsed.

When she returned to her home city, we were asked to take charge of her. On our first—and last —visit she greeted us with anger and abuse, using the vilest language we have heard—up to that time we thought the lumbermen of the Northwest were without peers in that line. We let her talk herself out, gave some advice and politely withdrew. We told the mother to call another doctor, that it would only harm her to have another visit from us since she seemed to think she had a grievance against us.

So the mother called the old family physician. The young lady treated him as she dealt with us, but he did not take her abuse in patience and silence, but shouted at her, "My God, young woman, don't you know that you are rotten through and through?"

She turned livid with rage, and toppled over—dead.

The end of the story we had from her mother, when she called on us to thank us for what we had done, also for what we had attempted to do for her daughter.

Yes, the emotions can and do kill, for some of them are as destructive as a tornado; and the depressing emotions can and do produce disease. Then the question arises, what are these emotions?

The most powerful are rage, shock, and intense fear. But there are many others: Worry is the child of fear, a weak emotion, but very destructive because it is almost constantly present in many lives; with fear and worry comes mental depression, which pulls down physical health. Anxiety and apprehension result from fear, worry and depression. And then there is that black emotion, self-pity, which wrecks many lives, for when it rules, balance is lost, and it drives away insight, deep understanding and vision. All centers in self and the cry is, "The world is against me." The real trouble is that the individual is against himself and the world, and this engenders unkindness and ill will. Jealousy and envy are other evil emotions; doubt condemns many to an inferior life. All of these emotions if much entertained cause disease.

All of these emotions if much entertained give rise to that great evil, tension, usually and wrongly called nervous tension. The right term is mental tension, for it is the mind that is in turmoil, the emotional part of the mind; and such turmoil upsets the rational or thinking part of the mind so it is unable to think straight and do good work.

So tension, or strain, or stress, prevents satisfaction in living, the greatest success in work, and it produces disease. It is easy to recognize tension, for it creates a tightening up of many parts of the body. It is felt in the neck, in the shoulders, in the chest and the abdomen—not necessarily in all of these places by the same individual. On examination, a doctor usually finds the arms much too stiff and unyielding—they are tightened up. So are the abdominal muscles, and worse still the delicate little muscles in the intestines, and that in the end causes constipation—a prominent cause of rheumatism and arthritis. We look upon tension as the greatest cause of arthritis, for it so upsets the whole body that it becomes increasing toxic, and the toxic state is the basis of diseases of all kinds.

HOW TO OVERCOME TENSION

First do a little evaluation of yourself: "I am one in billions on this little planet Earth. The earth is one in a family of planets trailing the Sun, our Day Star, in its orbit in the Milky Way. The Sun is an average star, in the billions of stars that make up the Milky Way. And the Milky Way is only one galaxy among the multitudes of known galaxies, each with billions of stars and no one knows how many planets, some of which probably have smarter and better looking inhabitants than earthly humanity.

"And I live in two great realities which I am unable to understand, infinity and eternity; lacking comprehension of these great totalities, I think of myself as living in time and space, on which my limited mind can set limits, and measure in hours and miles.

"Compared to the known galaxies, this Earth of ours is hardly a grain of sand. So from the physical standpoint, I can not be too important. If I crave importance, I can manifest it only in the mind and spirit. To do that I need much inner serenity."

An evaluation like that makes it easy to go on and get into a balanced mental habit, so as to use the thinking mind and direct the emotions to live satisfactorily, think and work to advantage and thus be successful, and at the same time build health (instead of building disease, as one does when dominated by fear, worry, depression and anxiety). Here are some of the steps to take to build the best of life and health possible:

MENTAL HEALTH BUILDING

1 "I shall give myself good care, and then forget myself in work or play, in their proper proportion."

2 "I shall not take myself as an individual so seriously, but shall be serious and sincere about my work."

3 "When my emotions are upset, I am unable to think clearly and act in the best way, so from now

on I am working for inner calmness, for serenity
and tranquility of mind. That is, when upsetting
and tensing emotions like fear, worry and anxiety
try to master me, I shall replace them with constructive, tranquilizing thoughts and emotions.
This I can do because I have directing power and
I have will power."

4 But what are the positive thoughts and emotions? The positive thoughts are the ones that come
in a calm state of mind, with the mind working
in confidence, in constructive, uplifting, upbuilding ways, looking for good results not only for self
but for others. The positive or constructive emotions are also tranquil ones, and the fundamental
ones are: Self-confidence, deep understanding of
self and others with a charitable outlook, good will,
hope and faith; employ these thoughts and emotions, and the essential courage grows and develops. If you believe in God, make your faith so abid-
ing, so innate, so indwelling that it drives away all
personal fears, worries, depressions, anxieties and
apprehensions. That is what flawless faith in God
can do, but if there is a flaw or doubt in this faith
—well, then there is no faith.

5 Suppose your disease-building emotions are
fear and worry; then say to yourself: "Fear and
worry produce turmoil in my mind, so I cannot
think right; they take charge of me and run me,
and then my work suffers; I feel badly and tense
up, and this upsets my digestion and creates tox-

ins within my body, and eventually the fear and worry help to build disease. I refuse to live under this tyranny, so I place faith and confidence where fear has been manifesting and then my worry vanishes. Whatever my depressive emotions have been, I replace them with constructive or positive emotions, and with the knowledge that when I do right, many good things will come my way."

6 "But I also realize that I cannot remake my thoughts and emotional directions at once, so I shall persist, no matter how long it takes."

7 When discouragement comes, always remember, "I can and I will." That is a pretty good slogan, is it not?

And then add this bit of truth to your philosophy of life: "All who are active, responsible and live the average length of years have their crosses and their losses; so I will have mine and meet them like an adult."

Not only study these truths over until they become a part of your thoughts and feelings, but act them out in your life, and you will see the change.

CASE HISTORIES CITED

How do human beings act when they meet adversity? Many do so with courage, as all adults should; too many try to avoid and evade difficulties, and get into trouble, for the right way is to face life with courage; and so many just go emotional when they encounter unusual difficulties. Let us illustrate:

Twenty years ago a woman who was ill both physically and emotionally consulted us. Her physical ills soon began to clear up; at the same time we were training her in meeting her human relationships so they would not keep her upset; this included relationships with relatives and in-laws. She learned to try to do her best, and trust what she could not do to God; she learned that some difficulties are a part of the game of living, so they should be faced calmly; she learned to think and express so as to have inner tranquility most of the time; she learned to meet the odds and ends of life, not as worries, but in the spirit of confidence. She has done wonderfully well in the intervening twenty years, even when she lost two of those who were nearest and dearest to her within a few months. And now she wants to be sure that she is on the correct road of physical, emotional and rational health for the rest of her life. A wise woman!

Yesterday we saw an arthritic woman who early in our relationship as patient and physician made a very great gain in her contest with arthritis. And then she stopped gaining—which is contrary to our experience. We have known for some time that there is a lack of harmony among the men in her family—the same old stupid impasse where the son or sons say that father is an old fogy and the father points to his success and stubbornly clings to the claim that the details that brought success thirty or more years ago are good enough; and then contention about it not only at business but at home.

This has upset the mother; she has felt bad about it, and it has sunk in, to her injury—she has not had the internal peace needed to overcome arthritis. As she can do nothing about this with her stubborn men, we tried to show her how to pay less and less attention to this state of affairs and not let it sink in; to remember that at heart the husband and sons esteem each other. In other words, she must not let the arthritis overcome her because the men in her family were having foolish spats, something that often happens when the son or sons go into the family business with their father. The whole thing could be solved with ease if the father would give the sons a little more freedom, a little more authority, as they make good, and if the sons would remember that after all, "Dad is a pretty good old scout." Yes, these are some of the considerations that go into the conquest of arthritis. Here is a sentence spoken by this arthritic mother, "Always, when they quarrel, my arthritis grows worse." Certainly, upset emotions worsen the arthritis.

Let us tell you another incident, this time involving disease of a father and a son. The father had not been strong for years. Whenever he was run down, he became afflicted with serious disease. Finally he had to spend too much time in bed, sometimes be-

ing unable to go to his place of business. He had
an adult son, and the plan for years was that father
and son were to do business together. But the son
held back—his stay in the army had adversely affected his health.

Finally father and son came to see us. We could
find no physical reason for the father's serious illness, but he had worried and fretted so much about
the son's absence from the business that he was as
tense and taut as a bow at the shooting point. This
made him ill, and the father's constant insistence
had made the son so antagonistic that he could not
talk to his father in the right way and spirit; his
speech became increasingly rapid and high pitched
until he reached the point where he was too keyed
up to speak. The father and son were on high tension with each other, so there was no meeting of
reasoning minds, merely the friction of destructive
emotions. It was so easy to see the reason the father
was ill and the son unhappy.

So we talked like a Dutch uncle to the father
showing him that he was too insistent and persistent, trying to dominate in the matter: we called to
his attention that even though he was carrying on
the business with the hope and idea of turning it
over to the son, he had to give the young man the
right of individuality, the right to make some wrong
decisions, the right to make some mistakes. When
the son realized that we were not going to reproach
him, it became easy to talk with him on a rational,

friendly level. We told him that as the business was to be a big fact in his future, his economic support, he could hardly blame his dad for wanting him to show present interest. We called his attention to the fact that he could start with his father for two or three or four hours a day, that he could stand that as easily as working full time in an office for someone else. When the son stated his case against the father, he grew increasingly tense and rapid and high-pitched, finally being unable to speak.

So we told him how to prevent this: "If you start to tighten up, immediately lower your voice and keep it deep; at the same time speak slowly, even more slowly than you do ordinarily in your calm moments; this gives you full control of yourself, full control of the English language which you use so well."

And finally we told him, in low, measured words: "We do not ask you to join your father; we do not say it is your duty, but we ask you just one thing, please tell your father within the next few days what you will do and when, for this waiting without decision is keeping him ill." This is what the father was after, but he had tried to force the issue. The son replied, "I am going into the business and will say so at the family meeting on Monday."

The change in the father's appearance was pleasant to see, and father and son left our office in friendly spirit.

We tell this in detail for this is the way psychology, or psychiatry, or the understanding of the mind, is employed to overcome disease and build good human relationship; it is largely a matter of replacing upset emotions with good will and straight thinking. When well done it builds better health, greater satisfaction or happiness, and more success.

Some say they are unable to change the emotional pattern, for they were born depressive or worrisome or fearful. This is a mistake. If we desire and will to change for the better, we can do it at any time in life.

First, we have directive or guiding power of the mind, so we can choose and develop the kind of mental patern we desire; we can go in the direction of mental-emotional turmoil, tension and depression, or we can choose confidence, tranquility and hopefulness. The basic determination is the direction or attitude of mind: As we direct or guide the mind, so the personality follows.

Thoughts are magnets that attract in kind.

So it is up to each one of us to direct the mind so it will flow in a constructive, upbuilding channel of thought. Of course, no reasonable person expects a human being to be perfect in this matter, but the important thing is for the mind to be constructive and hopeful most of the time. This is the health-building way.

The majority start a project with a will, in any walk of life, but so many lose interest when they find how much time and work it requires to attain the goal. It is so in arthritis: Some graduate into health, but too many quituate into chronic rheumatism and arthritis. It takes persistence and will power to win in the conquest of rheumatic and arthritic diseases.

WILL POWER

What is will power? It is a gift implanted in every human being; it is innate in all normal babies, for although they probably do not have it reasoned out, they have the will to live; as they grow and flourish, the will is channeled into various directions. But what is the will or will power?

It is a choosing, a deciding, a determining on a way of action or expression, with the stability to stay with the choice. To accomplish what is above average in life, this exertion of the will is essential; we have to adhere to our purpose until we accomplish or win. If we give up, we fail, whether it be a project in business, in professional work, in service, or in overcoming disease.

Arthritis is both insistent and persistent after it is well established; so we must be determined, we must use will power to overcome it. It is so easy to swallow some medicine or have some injections, but the right living in body and mind that brings lasting results in overcoming arthritis is sometimes a little difficult. It requires persistent following of the laws of Nature. It is those who cultivate will power and exert it who win out. And what a victory over the greatest crippler among diseases!

It requires the "I-can-and-will" spirit.

Those who permit fear, worry, depression and anxiety to rule their lives generally lose the fight with rheumatic disease, especially with arthritis.

Those who build up confidence, hope, faith, and good will, and at the same time live hygienically, generally conquer arthritis, and thus have a body that is a good instrument for mind and spirit.

I can and I will!

4 Obesity and Arthritis

Not all stout persons become rheumatic or arthritic, but when the body is too heavy it is so much easier to become ill. Stoutness smoothens the path for diabetes, Bright's disease, sciatica, hepatitis, various heart diseases, arteriosclerosis with high blood pressure (hypertension), and many other ills to enter the body; and stoutness is a direct invitation to rheumatism and arthritis to make themselves at home.

The truth is that after the age of forty, overweight is one of the greatest threats to human health. There are many reasons for this, and we shall give the most important ones.

Overweight, stoutness, fatness and obesity are four words for the same thing in varying degrees. All of them interfere with the circulation of the fluids of the body, for they crowd the blood-vessels and in this way hinder somewhat the free flow of the blood and lymph—the fat presses on the lymph channels too. When you realize that partial stagnation of the vital fluids is partial death, and that complete stagnation is physical death, you can realize also how vital it is to avoid stoutness.

Obesity is also a mechanical block to the freedom of the physical tissues and organs. The muscles are slowed down; the heart and the lungs, vital organs, are so oppressed by fat that upon extra effort the heart has to beat too hard and the lungs puff and pant. This means that stoutness reduces vital capacity.

And obesity shortens life, as the insurance statistics have conclusively shown. How often does the fat boy win the foot race? How often does the fat man win an endurance contest of any kind? They lose out in the race and contest of life too, for their years are shorter in the land—certainly, an occasional stout individual lives long, but it is the slender ones who set the fine records.

There is also a chemical reason for the inferior showing, in the race of life, of the obese. With the excessive fat they carry they have much toxic matter stored in the tissues. This toxic matter lowers living capacity and helps to produce disease; this is so true that we have repeatedly said that autointoxication is the basic cause of all disease; this toxicity leads to diseases of chronic degeneration, and we can so classify long-lasting arthritis and rheumatism.

But why do men and women grow stout? Why is overweight so common after the age of thirty or forty years? The answer is so simple. We wish men and women would take it to heart: It is because overeating is a common habit in this land of plenty.

During childhood and the teens the appetite is naturally keen because the body needs not only fuel and material for repairing the body; but much food is needed for growth, which implies added weight; also, the activity within the body is much greater during the first twenty years of life than at any other time. The result is that men and women attain the ages of twenty and even twenty-five with a keen appetite, and where food is plentiful they generally eat too much; because they are so active early in life, the penalty for overeating is not too great at this time (except in infancy, when it wreaks havoc).

However, at the age of thirty years or earlier, the young adult should realize this basic truth: "I quit growing some years ago, and my cells are no longer as active as they were in the teens and early twenties, so I should reduce my food intake, and more especially I should eat less of oils, fats, starches and all sweet foods." This realization seldom comes, and much disease from overeating is the result.

The food we need nourishes us and gives us strength.

The food we eat in excess of our needs builds disease and shortens life.

So the problem is to eat in such a way that the food helps us to have health, not disease; and one part of this problem is to avoid overeating.

But how is this done? We shall give you some important pointers to help you not only to remain slender, but healthful as well.

First, remember that if a man or woman is normal, his weight or hers between the ages of twenty-five and thirty years is the normal weight and should not go up later in life. For years it has been looked upon as natural and even desirable to fall into weight with the years. This is a mistake, for overweight is always an invitation to disease. Furthermore, the weights that physicians have been using as standard are wrong; they are based on insurance tables, showing that human beings gain weight as the decades roll on, being heavier in the thirties than in the twenties, still heavier in the forties, still gaining in the fifties and remaining too heavy in the sixties.

This is what has happened, and what has been looked upon as normal and desirable. But it is neither normal nor desirable; it is the result of overeating, after full growth has been attained, which is at the age of twenty-one in women and twenty-five in men, approximately.

So here is another important point: After the age of full growth, slowly reduce the food intake, eating a little less in the latter twenties than in the teens; still less in the thirties, and continue to decrease the food intake a little both in the forties and in the fifties. By doing this the weight is kept down and the figure remains slender—and this is a great aid in maintaining health and attaining long life.

We must here emphasize that the body needs less and less food, with the advancing years. The cells are not so active as they were in youth, and the rule is that the body is not put to as vigorous action in the middle years and afterwards as it was in early life. Moderation in eating is a key to maintaining good health, and thus preventing arthritis. Surely, it is as important to prevent disease as it is to overcome it.

But the difficulty is that an arthritic in the forties, or older, is too often overweight. Then what is he to do?

There are many who advocate exercises to overcome arthritis. However, many arthritics are too painful to exercise much. Besides, it is well known that exercising increases the appetite, and that often results in additional poundage. Also, overexercise of arthritic joints tends to make them more painful, with increase of the disease.

The surest way to reduce is to control the eating, taking more of lighter foods, such as fruits and vegetables, and less of the heavy foods, such as oils and fats, sugars and sweets, and starches, at the same time using salt very moderately.

11 POINTERS FOR REDUCING AT HOME

Here are some pointers about reducing that any human being can practice in his own home, and lose weight:

1 Omit from the food plan all oils, and all dressings made with oils, such as mayonnaise, Russian and French dressings. Also avoid oily fruits, such as the avocado and olives.

2 Do not eat any fatty meats or fish, such as pork, fatty beef, the fatty parts of lamb, tuna, salmon, whitefish and bluefish, mackerel and herring. Take the leaner meats and fish—not the greasy ones.

3 Let alone all fried foods, all greasy cooking, all thickened gravies or sauces, whether for meats or fish or vegetables or starches.

4 Use cream seldom and sparingly; do not put it in any drinks and a small amount once a week in the meal should be the top limit while reducing. Let the butter portions be small.

5 Be sparing in your intake of starches, such as bread and potatoes, remembering that an ounce of bread is twice as fattening as an ounce of potatoes. Do your best to cut the starch intake in two.

6 Here is a very fine aid in reducing—do not take any food made of grains or flour in your dinner —no bread, no biscuits, no toast, no breadstuffs of any kind in the dinner, please. You do not need the grains or cereals in the dinner, for you generally have meat or fish with plenty of vegetables and some potato in this meal. This hint is good for everybody, even though they have no arthritis.

7 Omit all white sugar—this is also good for all, for white sugar is a dead food that can only harm the human body. Even omit such good sweets as honey, maple sugar, brown sugar (often called raw sugar), and those excellent sweets—raisins, figs, dates, sweet prunes, and ripe bananas—while reducing.

And by all means do not take the dessert sweets —cake, cookies, pies, puddings and ice cream. These are too rich and fattening to eat while reducing; nor are they good foods for arthritics. This is true even if the arthritics are slender; certainly, some of those who have arthritis are thin.

Now we have told you some of the things not to do. Please pay attention to the things that you should do:

8 Let at least three-fourths of your breakfast, by

weight, consist of unsweetened cooked or raw
fruits, including berries and melons, but avoiding
the fattening fruits—raisins, figs, dates, prunes, ripe
bananas, melons and avocados. The less bread or
toast or cereal, the better. An all fruit breakfast is
best while reducing.

9 Let your lunch consist by weight of over two-
thirds of garden vegetables, cooked and raw, but
either avoid or take seldom and sparingly of parsnips, corn, beets and lima beans; take carrots and
peas only once a week while reducing. The rest of
the vegetables you may consume freely, except
rhubarb, which is so full of oxalic acid that it is not
good for anyone—the green parts of this plant are
so full of oxalic acids that they have caused direct
poisoning when consumed as greens. Tomatoes are
good, but they are so full of acid that they should
be taken sparingly in arthritis. You may be told not
to take spinach or other leafy greens, but they are
good for you—help yourself. If they contain oxalic
acid it is in such tiny amounts that they will never
hurt you.

10 Let your dinner consist of about three-
fourths of vegetables by weight, raw and cooked.

11 If you wish dessert, take fruit, cooked or raw,
no sweetening or cream added.

If you are overweight, whether rheumatic, arthritic or not, and get into the spirit of the matter,
following these directions to the letter, you will

lose weight and not only strengthen your health but lengthen your life.

For obesity decreases health, induces disease and shortens life. Obesity is in and of itself a disease, so why entertain this enemy?

5 How Constipation Cripples Arthritics

Constipation is not the only cause of crippling arthritis, but it is one of the most prominent of the physical causes; and arthritis cripples more human beings than any other disease. Constipation is also one of the outstanding factors in producing rheumatism. The truth is that it is one of the great evils of civilized life; it should not be tolerated; it need not be tolerated, for reasonable precautions in the living mode prevent this filthiest of ills.

Please let us explain: The waste expelled from the bowels is rather moist, so there is no hardness, no lumpiness in it; the moisture carries in solution such matters as sulphuric acid, phenol (carbolic acid), skatol, indol, bacterial wastes and other poisons. When constipation is permitted, much of the moisture, with its poisonous products, finds its way back into the blood and lymph, and is distributed to the whole body, causing many ills, such as pimples, headaches, eczema, colds, bronchitis, nephritis, rheumatism and arthritis. What a price to pay for carrying poisonous waste around within the body, after it should have been expelled!

Some physicians advise the public that it does not matter whether the bowels function daily. They could not be more wrong if they tried, and those who accept this advice pay dearly for so doing. To remain healthy, the body has to be clean within, and there is no cleanliness when the intestine is constipated. The waste should be fully expelled from the colon at least once a day, and the movement should be complete and satisfactory, with no lumpiness in any part of it. Those who are able to have two movements a day are fortunate, and three good movements daily are favorable to health.

OBEY THE CALLS OF NATURE

One of the chief causes of constipation may seem odd to many, for it is neglecting the call of Nature. The normal colon notifies the individual that there is waste to cast out in the lower bowel. This call should be heeded at once, for so long as it is heeded it remains clear and unmistakable. But if the policy is to delay increasingly, the call comes more seldom and with less clarity, and finally it does not come —that means constipation. And constipation means disease unless much ado is practiced to get the bowels to cleanse themselves.

Too limited water drinking, wrong eating, too little physical activity and what we call nervous tension are other causative factors. But here we must explain what will almost surely be recorded elsewhere—what we call nervous tension is not nervous in origin; it is mental tension for it comes only to those who are disturbed in thoughts and emotions; in other words it is mental tension—lack of mental adjustment.

Elsewhere we shall go into detail about the correct feeding to overcome rheumatism and arthritis. Fortunately, that kind of eating helps to prevent constipation; it also helps to restore the intestines to normal functioning, if it is still possible. But if the bowels are neglected for many years, they become irritated and sometimes so scarred that they are unable to normalize—we are thankful to say that often the most unpromising colon begins to function well again, even after years of neglect.

Please let us call to your attention the fact that normal water drinking and eating freely of fresh fruits and fresh vegetables, cooked or raw, are among the most powerful physical factors in overcoming constipation. These three—water, fruits and vegetables—are our chief remedies in many ills, including arthritis and rheumatism. The victim of these two ills should eat freely of fruits for breakfast, and take large servings of vegetables

in the lunch and in the dinner, having cooked vegetables in both meals, and raw vegetables or salad,
at least once, better twice daily.

MENTAL TENSION AND CONSTIPATION

But how does mental tension help to cause constipation? By producing physical tension. When the
mind tightens or tenses, so do the muscles of the
body and the nerves. Then the muscles do not act
so effectively. One may not notice this in the great
muscles of the body, such as we find in the arms,
legs and trunk; but if the delicate muscles in the
intestines underwork, the regular motion of the
intestines—peristalsis—decreases in effectiveness;
and then the forward propulsion of the waste in
the bowel becomes subnormal, and that is constipation. The great forward movement of the waste,
known as mass peristalsis, normally takes place two
or three times a day; this is essential to full cleanliness of the intestines; this precious function may
be lost because of tension originating in the mind.

The remedy is to calm the mind, and to work and
live in confidence. However, this is such a big subject that the principles of the healthful use of the
mind will be laid down in another chapter.

We regret to say that some who give advice to
the public tell those who listen to them that there
is no need of drinking water unless thirsty. In the-

ory this seems good, but in practice it is dangerous counsel, for those who drink too little water become toxic, and toxicity is a cause of disease. It is so easy to get the habit of limiting the water drinking, especially if one takes coffee, and tea, which are drugged drinks, or orange juice, or milk, or soup, which are liquid foods.

During every second of life, the body produces poisonous waste, and there is only one substance that carries this toxic matter out of the body—water. No matter what other liquids are imbibed or eaten, we need water. So one important rule for preventing or overcoming constipation is to drink plenty of water. A small person should drink at least five glasses (forty ounces) of water per day; a large individual should take more.

Let us repeat that those who drink enough water, eat freely of fruits and vegetables, obey the calls of Nature, maintain reasonable physical activity, and at the same time keep the mind hopeful and constructive, do not become constipated.

FIVE RULES FOR OVERCOMING CONSTIPATION

But if constipation is already present, as it is in the great majority of rheumatics and arthritics, what is one to do? The key is in the preceding paragraph, but this is so important that we shall enumerate the steps to take:

1 Make a habit, if a small person, to drink at least five glasses of water every day, and we mean water; if you had to pay a high price for each glass, you would appreciate it. It is good to rinse the mouth on first arising, and then drink one or two glasses of water any temperature desired except that chilled or iced water is not good at any time— yes, comfortably hot water is good in the morning. And then drink the rest of your quota during the day, but avoid drinking during meals. You may drink at the beginning or end of meals, or between meals.

2 Begin the breakfast with a large serving of fruit (this includes melons and berries), cooked or raw but add no white sugar; and instead of eating highly refined white breadstuffs and cereals, take the whole grain products, such as whole wheat toast, or a cereal made of whole corn, or whole wheat, and this means that all of the germ is kept in the food.

3 In the lunch have at least one large dish of cooked vegetable and maybe a raw vegetable, avoiding all fried and devitalized foods. More will be told in the chapter or chapters devoted to foods, in this book. In the dinner have a raw vegetable salad and at least one large serving of cooked vegetables; for dessert eat fruit.

4 Do your best to establish a certain time, better two times, each day for the bowels to function. Inasmuch as food acts as a stimulant to the diges-

tive tract, the best times are soon after meals. So we suggest going to the bathroom within thirty or forty minutes after breakfast, also within the same time limit after dinner, and give the intestines the chance to act. This is a wonderful help in establishing a normal habit, but one has to be persistent.

5 If the body is not active enough, and if the work is not of such a nature that the intestinal cavity contracts and expands often during the day, some simple exercises should be taken. Brisk walking is fine; when the weather is good, it is perhaps the best of exercises; the best indoor exercise of which we know for this purpose is the deep-knee bend (squatting), beginning with five or six at a time and working up gradually until squatting at least twenty times per day. Lying flat on a mat on the floor and exercising the legs with the bicycle movement is also good; and so it is to throw the arms around the thighs and rock back and forth on the curved back. Another simple exercise is to stand up and pretend to pull the abdominal wall upward and backward under the ribs, and then relax; repeat about twenty times after getting used to it.

Please remember, if not used to exercises, that it is best to begin with a few, and gradually increase to the right number. This avoids extreme soreness from overusing unused muscles. There are many other exercises good for constipation.

6 Avoid habitual fear, worry, depression, anxiety—yes, avoid as much as possible all depressing and tensing emotions. Replace them with self-confidence, with kindness, with good will, and with hope, expecting and looking for your share of the good things of life. This relaxes the intestinal muscles, so the intestinal motility normalizes. Surely, we shall have much more to say about benefiting by wholesome thoughts and emotions.

But suppose you do all of these things and the bowels refuse to function of and by themselves! Then it is necessary to resort to artificial aid.

Some need only the mild stimulation of a glycerine suppository for the desired result. Use that when it is necessary.

Some need only a small enema, the amount injected with a baby syringe. In that case use plain water, or water containing a little table salt, or water made opaque with clean castile soap.

Others need a larger enema, one or two quarts of tepid water, plain or treated as the small enema is. Do not use more water than needed, and if the bowels move well by themselves, let them alone. But in rheumatism and arthritis a good movement of the bowels every day is a must.

We had one patient who had been afflicted with constipation more than twenty years. His own words were, "I have not had a natural movement in twenty years." He said he was tired of laxatives and cathartics, and wished to be normal again. So we resorted to the tapering enema, beginning with two quarts of tepid water; each week the water was reduced so that at the end of three months he was having good results with one quart daily; in two additional months he was down to a cup each day, and a few days later he stopped using the enema, and the bowels functioned without artificial aid.

Of course, he drank his quota of water, he ate right, he took exercises that expanded and contracted the abdomen; as a result, he overcame another annoying disease while he conquered the constipation. This kind of conquest requires patience and persistence, but the patient thought it was more than worth while to function normally once more.

LAXATIVES AND CATHARTICS

What about laxatives and cathartics? Most of them are bad because with the passing of time larger and larger doses are required, and this means that when relying on them, the patient grows increasingly constipated. In emergencies they may be used, and occasional flushing of the bowel with a purgative, like citrate of magnesia followed with the drinking of hot lemon water, may be an advantage; but laxatives or cathartics should not become a habit. Among the mildest of laxatives are milk of magnesia and cascara sagrada; the latter has the advantage of calling for little or no increase in the dosage—I have had patients who gave me the history of using cascara for ten or twenty or more years without increasing the dose.

What about the herbal laxatives on the market? Most of them contain senna, which is a rather powerful laxative or cathartic, and the fact remains that those who are able to regain normal bowel functioning will fare best if they do so.

Most remedies lose their effectiveness after being used a while, so those who use them find it good policy to have several, and change from time to time.

There are the unfortunate ones who are unable to regain normal function, for the intestines refuse to respond to natural measure. These will have to depend on artificial aids. After long constipation, some intestines become fibrosed (scarred), after which the return to normal is difficult, and sometimes impossible.

But fortunately, the majority can improve, many of them to the point of normalcy. So the best policy is to make a persistent try for this desirable condition.

Are there any laxative foods? In general, the fruits and vegetables tend to normalize the bowels.

Roughage is a mechanical stimulant, but should not be overdone. Prunes, figs, pears, spinach and stewed onions have a reputation as laxative, and for some they work, but not for all. Hygienic living is the best way.

6 Rheumatic Fever

Rheumatic fever is mostly a disease of children, more often seen among girls than in boys, in which the sensitiveness, soreness and pain are often extreme; there is usually multiple arthritis with a great tendency to carditis, more especially endocarditis which may leave valvular damage. The arthritis clears up, but leaves the individual susceptible to arthritis later in life, unless he lives so hygienically that he avoids toxicity in adulthood. It is generally preceded by a sore throat, and more especially a streptococcus sore throat; the tendency is for the disease to recur, and the more attacks there are, the greater are the chances for permanent heart damage—leaking heart valves with accompanying murmurs.

If parents would stop pampering children, feed them right, but avoid overfeeding them, and take the correct steps when the throat becomes sore,

they would prevent this disease, and that is what
we wish to stress in this chapter.

First, there is no need for multiple attacks. In
over forty years, not one of our patients has had
even a second attack of rheumatic fever. Why?
Because the parents have adopted a wholesome
mode of caring for their children. We believe rheumatic fever is impossible if the children are raised
so they stay sweet and clean throughout—sweet
and clean blood, muscles, nerves, glands, organs,
etc. Yes, this necessitates clean intestines.

SYMPTOMS AND PREVENTION

How does rheumatic fever start? Generally as a
sore throat. The child is usually cross and finicky.
Observant parents easily realize that the child
neither looks right nor acts right; it has the feverish look even before the fever is apparent; it loses
interest in many good foods, although it will eat
fancy junk, containing plenty of white sugar.

What should be done? Such a child should be
given a purge, or at least a good enema—the purge
is better the first day—and put to bed; all feeding
should stop, liquid or solid; we mean exactly that,
for the food feeds the toxicity and the disease when
a child is preparing to become severely ill; when
no food is taken the body has a full chance to throw
off the disease. But water should be given freely,

at any temperature the child wishes while not eating; a little lemon juice may be added to the drinking water. If the child will not take lemon juice, give one or two small doses of your pet alkaline remedy daily—the best known one is sodium bicarbonate. Do this until the child brightens up and looks normal around the eyes and mouth, yes, do this until all signs of an impending sore throat leave. It does not take long, and may prevent a tragedy. Plenty of water, please, and be sure that the bowels move every day even if an enema is needed.

When we said to give no food, we meant exactly that: No broth, no milk, no soup, no custard—just put the child to bed for a few days, give plenty of water, keep the bowels clean and no food. Most of the children clear up beautifully on this plan in three or four or five days, but they have to be taken in hand before the fever begins to rage to get these results. It has always worked. Nature is wonderful —yes, Nature is grand! If we only have sense enough to heed her dictum not to give or take food when acute disease threatens, when we lose our normal appetite! Fixing tempting dishes for those who lose their appetites because they are threatened with acute disease is a terrible blunder.

When such children normalize, begin to give them fruit juice, then fruits, and vegetables, and milk and other good foods, but do not return them to devitalized foods—study the section on foods and cooking at the end of this book.

TREATMENT OF ESTABLISHED CASES

But suppose a child already has rheumatic fever. Then he also has a doctor, for it is far too disturbing for the family to attempt full care and responsibility. But we shall give something fundamental despite this fact.

Of course the patient is made easy; if terribly painful, the patient is handled in a sheet, and sponged daily, for that peculiar sour-sweet odor coming from the body is quite disagreeable; and either a mild laxative is given or the enema is used so the bowels will be well cleansed. If needed, cradles are used to hold up bedding.

But the most important thing is not to give any food, liquid or solid, so long as the fever lasts. This shortens the fever, clears up the arthritis (painful joints) sooner, and reduces the incidence of permanent heart damage.

Even cats and dogs know they should not eat when they have fever—it is pretty near time for homo sapiens—not always so sapient—to learn this and to apply this bit of life- and health-saving wisdom.

When the fever leaves, the child gradually returns to food, but the important thing is to eat wholesome foods that will help to prevent further attacks. This means that cake, cookies, pie, puddings, candies and all fried foods, all foods containing white flour and white sugar should be discontinued. It further means that the food plan should include plenty of fresh vegetables, cooked and raw, a large amount of fruit, and that the child should drink water freely, and learn to have a good free bowel movement daily—it is splendid for children to have two bowel movements each day.

Although rheumatic fever is hardly rheumatism, hardly arthritis, these ills are present, and every family should have the knowledge in this brief chapter. Rheumatic fever is more like a bacterial intoxication. The important thing is to prevent it if possible, and if it is present to treat it so it will not wreck the heart.

7 Gout

Gout is a uric acid intoxication of the body, with the tendency for a high level of uric acid retention in the blood, and generally a too low excretion of uric acid and its products (urates) in the urine. It is looked upon as constitutional and hereditary, but this we doubt. What is inherited, or rather acquired, is the wrong mode of living of the parents, and this upsets the constitution.

Gout is mostly a disease in men over forty years of age—women seldom have it. It may occur in various joints—seldom in hips, spine and shoulders—but over half of the time it manifests in the big toe. The affected joint becomes red, swollen and painful, and later it peels.

If the patient carries his toxic condition with him at all times, he may have sudden attacks. If he rids himself of the toxicity by living right, the attacks stop. If the gout is permitted to remain, deformity may follow, generally after repeated attacks.

In English literature gout has long been attributed to high living; and it is easy enough to confirm that it is caused by wrong living, especially wrong eating and drinking with deficient and delayed elimination.

On the whole, the treatment is the same as that for arthritis. But the uric acid angle needs special attention, and so do the acute attacks. These attacks may last for only a few days, or they may run on for weeks.

As the affected parts are so painful, rest is indicated, with the joint made comfortable—usually only one joint is affected. If this joint is in the big toe, it may be advisable to have the foot in a cradle, somewhat elevated, and it may be necessary to use much cotton batting to give comfort. Naturally, a professional person will be called, at least in the first attack, and he will show how such things are done.

NATURAL TREATMENT OF GOUT

The natural treatment is simple. Give a mild purgative, such as citrate of magnesia, to clear the waste out of the colon; give water freely; make the patient comfortable, and stop the intake of all solid food. Yes, stop giving all foods known as proteins, which are meat, fish, eggs, cheese and milk; stop giving all starches, which are principaly the cereals, including all breadstuffs, all foods made of flour, all of the breakfast cereals; stop giving all the sweets, meaning sugars of every kind, syrups, honey, molasses and of course all pies and cakes and puddings and cookies; stop giving all fats and oils—butter, olive oil and all of the oily dressings —stop using all oils. This you do until the patient is comfortable.

What is there left to eat? All the fresh fruits in the market, and all fresh and frozen vegetables in the market, and water to drink. And this is being generous, for the patient would be best treated by going on a water fast for three to five days, with a daily enema.

For breakfast have a glass of fruit juice, and one or two fresh fruits.

For lunch have some raw vegetable or vegetables, with or without a little salt, one or two cooked vegetables, and top off this meal with one fruit.

For dinner have a raw vegetable, or some mixed raw vegetables, and one or two cooked vegetables, with fruit for dessert.

If you so desire, a glass of fruit juice in the middle of the afternoon. It is best not to take more than two glasses of fruit juice per day during the painful stage which is so irksome, for large amounts of fruit acids may accentuate the pain.

And remember to drink six or more glasses of

water every day; also be certain that the bowels are well cleansed every day, even if an enema is needed for this purpose.

When the pain leaves, add first of all baked potato to the dinner; then have a little toast with the lunch; but take just fruit and juice for the breakfast, for a few weeks.

And then return to a food plan such as we have allowed in arthritis, in which we outline many menus, but with this exception:

In gout, protein is to be eaten only once a day until one is certain that the gouty tendency has left the system, until the high level of uric acid or urates no longer exists in the blood or the rest of the body.

In other words, take no milk, or cheese, or eggs or nuts either in the breakfast or in the lunch—and of course no meat or fish.

But have your one protein of the day in the dinner, omitting all pork and all beef. Yes, ham and bacon are pork, so they are to be off limits. For your dinner proteins select one of the following, and only one in a dinner, glass of milk, a serving of cottage cheese, one or two eggs, ocean fish, chicken, turkey, veal, or lamb—only one of these in a dinner, please; only one of these all day, please, until the gouty tendency is overcome.

The water drinking has much to do with vanquishing the gout.

Use fat very sparingly. Do not permit overweight, for that helps to invite gout to return. Get that weight down to normal and keep it so.

As for tea, coffee, tobacco and alcohol, they help the gout to maintain itself in the body; these indulgences should be discontinued. Wine and other liquors have long been blamed for the gout. It is true that uric acid stored in the body is given as the cause of gout, but this is not the only factor by any means. Gout is a disease of self-indulgence.

But the uric acid and its urates are so important in this disease that it is important to know that the uric acid and urates in the body are the results of burning proteins in the muscles and other tissues (oxidation). As the system contains an excess of these compounds, it is necessary to take proteins in great moderation, especially meat and fish and eggs.

Also, please remember that water is the compound that floats all the poisons out of the body, including uric acid and urates. So drink freely of water in gout.

8   The Rheumatic Diathesis

Years ago we heard much about rheumatic diathesis, tubercular diathesis, and other forms of
diathesis; this word is rather seldom heard now—it
means a state of body favorable to developing disease. There is both reality and fallacy back of this
idea.

There are conditions of body favorable to disease
formation; the toxic state, that is, the condition in
which the body is poisoned by its own retained
wastes, is such a reality. When a person is toxic he
can easily develop rheumatism or arthritis, or both;
but he can with equal facility become hypertensive
or a victim of heart disease, such as cardiac throm-
bosis or endocarditis. The toxic state is at the foundation of disease. Many think a little germ (bacte-
rium) comes along and creates a disease; or maybe
a virus produces a disease. However, those who
have healthy bodies have great resistance to dis-

ease influence, but those who are toxic easily fall victims of the bacteria or viruses. So it is most important to live hygienically for the purpose of having a healthy body that will not fall easy prey to every swarm of bacteria that comes along.

All who study the subject with logical care find it easy to understand that a healthy body resists disease, and a toxic body falls easy prey to various ills. But no one knows for sure why millions of Americans are the victims of rheumatism and arthritis, while even more millions are destroyed by the arterio-cardiac complex of diseases (high blood pressure with stroke and heart disease). Saying that disease attacks the weakest part of the body is probably expressing the truth, but it adds very little to understanding.

HOW CHILDREN ARE AFFECTED

Years ago we often heard about growing pains; this term is seldom used now for two reasons; there is less rheumatism among children than formerly because children now consume more of fruits and vegetables, and this produces a purer blood stream. So growing pains occur more seldom; growing pains were and are a form of rheumatism among the young. Growth is normal to a child and does not create pain.

If it should happen to your child, the remedy is very simple: Stop the white sugar intake and give the child more fruit; stop the white flour and white bread intake and give the child whole grain foods; increase the drinking of water; be sure the bowels are kept clean, and let the child have an abundance of fresh air and sunshine. Give plenty of fresh vegetables for lunch and for dinner.

As for the rheumatic diathesis, it is nothing but the toxic state. We shall deal with this under the heading of treatment in other chapters, so it will merely be discussed here for the purpose of adding to the reader's understanding.

The toxic condition comes about because of wrong physical living, poor elimination, and mental-emotional misdirection. In most households, white sugar is consumed in abundance, the average person getting about 100 pounds, maybe more, every year, if candy, cake, and sweetening of foods and drinks be added together. White sugar is a carbon food containing heat and energy units. But it has no health value; it is completely deprived of organic mineral salts and vitamins; and although sugar is a neutral food, it does lower the alkalinity of the body because the bicarbonates in the blood are used in eliminating the carbonic acid gas which is a byproduct of carbon oxidation in the muscles and other body structures. White sugar is the most impoverished food we have, and a source of toxicity from childhood onward.

White flour and the breadstuffs made therefrom
are not as bad as white sugar, but they are inferior
foods. The whole wheat kernel contains numerous
organic compounds called mineral salts; also many
vitamins; these are precious builders of health.
When the bran and the germ are removed, the laxative part of the grain is lost, and so are many of
the health values, for they reside mostly in the bran
and the germ. We have the inferior white starch
left; it is partly devitalized when it loses the bran
and the germ, and further so when the flour is
bleached.

DIATHESIS BUILDERS

And so it is that white breadstuffs, and all foods
made of white flour are inferior; they have lost so
much of their vitality that they add to the bodily
toxicity, and that is the same as saying that the
consumption of white sugar and white flour products is one causation of the rheumatic diathesis;
and rheumatism strongly tends to run into arthritis,
in time.

Another diathesis builder is frying. Frying is the
worst of all methods of cooking. Frying makes all
foods harder to digest, for it hardens the food with
hot fat, making it difficult for the digestive juices
to penetrate the pieces of food that enter the stomach; then the digestion suffers, and this results in

The Rheumatic Diathesis 75

the formation of inferior blood, which is unable to maintain or build healthy body tissues. Frying should be discontinued even by those who are healthy; it is imperative for rheumatics and arthritics to give up this mode of cooking, for it helps to build the toxicity that in turn causes arthritis.

Another reason for the toxicity that causes disease, including the rheumatic diathesis, is constipation, which parents permit to creep into the lives of their children, and which these children when adults further invite. We especially mention this here so we may call to your attention more than once the fact that constipation is a prominent cause of arthritis. More especially, we wish to emphasize that ignoring and neglecting the calls of Nature is the chief cause of constipation.

A normal child will have two bowel movements daily—certainly one movement a day, but two movements are more beneficial and natural in childhood. By promptly obeying the calls of Nature the function of quick elimination can be maintained, and this is a great factor in retaining health, in preventing disease. For if the waste is permitted to remain in the colon, the poisonous part residing in the moisture of that waste is reabsorbed into the blood and the lymph and that poisons the body; this means that such a person is intoxicated (poisoned) by his own wastes. That is, goes deeper and deeper into the autointoxication back of any

diathesis, which too often turns out to be rheumatic or arthritic.

Parents have the blessed privilege of teaching
their children about the importance of this function of prompt bowel elimination; about the fact
that by promptly obeying the calls of Nature, this
function is maintained; that this is a powerful factor in building the agility and strength that boys
so much desire, and the beauty so dear to the heart
of the girls. Yes, both the boys and the girls find
their studies easier when the bowels function fully
and well; and the boys are better at games and the
girls more attractive when the bowel function is
normal.

What about adults? They are more effective,
happier and healthier with normal bowel function, and this means more successful. And the
women maintain the loveliness of the skin, which
so enhances beauty, for many additional years.

Now we have told you some of the chief physical reasons for the rheumatic diathesis, which may
be called the toxic state or autointoxication. We
shall mention only one mental condition:

It is the depressive, destructive mental-emotional state. Human beings walk through life full of
fear; so they worry and they fret; they become de-
pressed and anxious; they are enchained with apprehension. As this pulls down the thinking mind
and the emotions, so it plays havoc with the digestion and the assimilation and helps to produce in-

ferior blood, ending with deteriorating body. Please study carefully the chapter dealing with the mind; also the chapter on constipation.

And by example and precept, teach your children to walk the path of life courageously; teach them to have confidence in themselves; teach them that they do best when they are calm and kind; teach them to have faith and hope—yes, teach them the constructive way of thinking and expressing.

And by all means, teach them that although life holds many fine things for those who work for them, there are troubles and difficulties in every life; when these arise, the greatest asset one has is to remain calm, confident and hopeful.

Not only teach this to the children, but tell it to yourselves, for this constructive attitude helps adults of all ages, as well as the boys and girls in their teens.

And please never whine, "But this is so difficult to do."

Remember, I can and I will. I have a backbone —no jellyfish am I.

II TREATMENT OF ARTHRITIS AND RHEUMATISM

9 Acute Rheumatoid Arthritis

Before we deal with rheumatoid arthritis, please let us discuss arthritis as a whole, and more about its classification. Arthritis simply means inflammation seated in one or more joints, and aside from mechanical arthritis, the disease is usually multiple; in bad cases all the joints of the arms, hands, legs and feet may be affected, although the disease is not as common in the shoulders and the hips as in smaller joints—one or many of the joints of the spine may also be involved.

Arthritis is usually classified according to its causation, and it would not be difficult to mention twenty or thirty forms of arthritis, but it would serve no useful purpose. Tubercular arthritis means that the tuberculosis bacillus is a part of the picture. Menopausal arthritis explains itself, but let us hasten to explain that the menopause does not cause arthritis in a healthy woman. Here are the chief forms of arthritis.

1 Rheumatoid arthritis, seen mostly in the hands where the joints are swollen; also present in the spinal joints where it is called rheumatoid spondylitis. Rheumatoid arthritis is seen far more frequently than any other form of arthritis. If permitted to continue it can easily render the joints useless, in time, and create deformities.

2 Degenerative arthritis, or chronic joint disease. In this class we have what is known as osteo-arthritis, which not only involves the joint structure but degeneration of the bones themselves; also hypertrophic arthritis, in which there is great enlargement of the affected parts.

3 Infective arthritis, which explains itself; bacteria associated with other diseases are present. And here we might include arthritis following debilitating diseases which have finally reduced the vitality until the joints become affected; there is also arthritis after the consumption of too many toxic drugs; and there is emotional arthritis, as in hysteria.

4 Traumatic arthritis is of course due to injury. In addition, arthritis can result from diseased nerves or from tumors, or neoplasms, as some of

these are called. And we are also discussing gout and rheumatic fever.

The fact is that when the body deteriorates, as it does with the years because conventional living modes tend to produce disease, arthritis too often occurs. It is frequently impossible to put one's finger on a certain causative factor and say this is it. But, barring accidents, we have always found a toxic body in arthritis.

SYMPTOMS OF RHEUMATOID ARTHRITIS

Rheumatoid arthritis is a case in point. It is usually defined as a chronic form of arthritis of unknown origin, affecting many joints, with accompanying weakness; its peculiarity is the formation of granulations in and about the joints; the result is pain, limitation of motion, deformity and sometime loss of all motion in one or more joints—this happens when the joints lime up and is known as ankylosis. Rheumatoid arthritis is also known as arthritis deformans, atrophic arthritis, proliferative arthritis and chronic infectious arthritis.

Why is this disease defined as chronic? Please read this with care, for it may save you much trouble. The fact is that it is acute in the beginning, but not "too troublesome" at first, as many a woman has told us. So most doctors see little of and seldom recognize it for what it is, the very first stages of recognizable arthritis.

Here is how it starts: A woman (sometimes it is a man) realizes some fine morning that her hands are clumsy, the fingers being a little stiff, but if she soaks the hands in hot water or does some work, the clumsiness and stiffness of fingers vanish for the day.

So she does nothing about it, even if the stiffness of fingers persists a week or two.

There is a tendency for the condition to remit; but the stiffness of fingers returns, and then there is some soreness. As the morning goes on the condition clears up, but a little later than formerly.

Still she does nothing about it.

There is another remission and she thinks the trouble has vanished. But it returns. This time it is not only stiffness and soreness, but a little pain has been added. However, as she busies herself the condition goes away, leaving her hands easy for the rest of the day. But it stays longer, maybe most of the forenoon.

And still she does nothing about it.

The condition comes and goes and finally she notices that in addition to stiffness of fingers, soreness and pain, there is puffiness of the fingers. And finally a little joint reddens and swells; she probably does nothing about that either, and then the corresponding joint on the opposite hand reddens and swells. By this time a prudent woman will surely consult a physician, you think. But not always so. Some women wait until many joints are inflamed, until the condition diagnoses itself as arthritis. The truth is that it was arthritis from the very start of stiffened fingers and clumsiness of hands.

At this stage it is unbelievably easy and simple to stop the disease in its tracks, clear it up and make the patient safe from arthritis for life, if she has the will and the desire to live healthfully, so as to maintain a wholesome body.

But why do not women heed the warnings as they see these acute attacks grow worse? Because there are remissions, and then they deceive themselves to think they will have no more; when an attack lets up they say to themselves that this is the last one. Self-deception is often worse than fibbing to others.

And because the patients generally stay away during the acute stage of rheumatoid arthritis, many doctors think of it as only a chronic disease, and dictionaries so define it; the truth is that there are usually many acute attacks of this disease, before the chronic form takes place.

And it is obvious that if the acute form of rheumatoid arthritis were correctly treated and cleared up, there would be no chronic rheumatoid arthritis.

There is acute rheumatoid arthritis that is almost explosive in its severity, with great pain, swelling, and limitation of motion. But always there is either great toxicity or some bad upset before this can take place. In this severe kind of arthritis, use hot or cold applications—whichever gives greater comfort; clean the bowels with enemas or mild alkaline laxatives, and keep them clean; the patient belongs in bed, and if very painful, it may be well to use cradles for the affected parts so the bedding will not become a burden; and most important, stop all eating, liquid and solid, until the pain recedes; but drink very freely of water, with or without a little lemon juice. With this treatment the pains soon leave, and then the food plans will be plenty of vegetables twice a day; plenty of fruit for breakfast, and solid foods in moderation, avoiding all devitalized foods—see the last section of this book.

TREATMENT OF ACUTE RHEUMATOID ARTHRITIS

We repeat, when a patient comes in the early stages of acute rheumatoid arthritis, it is easy to bring about a recovery, a permanent recovery if the patient wishes. Having had a rather extensive reputation in arthritis work for at least four decades, many such patients have consulted us. Never was there any difficulty about the recovery in this early stage when the patient cooperated.

Perhaps the best way to inform you what is to

be done in a condition of this kind is to summarize
the way we have dealt with our personal patients.
First we size up the conditions, as to state of body,
past history and habits. Up to date we have found
the living habits adverse to health, in every instance; and furthermore, we have found the patient too acid (toxic)—in every instance. So we sit
down and explain matters to the patient, usually
in this way, which is as near the average as we can
make it:

"Health depends on the daily habits of living.
There are certain natural laws that rule over us;
if we observe these laws and practice them, or
closely approximate them, we maintain health or
rebuild it, if health has already been lost. If we
disregard these rules—most persons say break these
rules or laws—we build disease. Incidentally, we
have not the power to break the laws of Nature,
for these rules are absolute; we can disregard them,
and then we break our own health.

"You have taken too much coffee, and perhaps
too much tea; you have had your cocktails much
too often, and you have smoked about fifteen cigarettes a day. All of these have helped to poison or
intoxicate you, and have helped to make your
body so acid that health has abdicated—your fingers and hands are the result of this intoxication.
So this is what we recommend: It is easy enough
to stop the tea and all alcohol, so please do that;
for a young woman it is also easy to reduce the cof-

fee drinking to one cup a day, so take your cup of breakfast coffee and no more that day. As for the cigarettes, if you have good will power you can stop smoking right now—some of our patients have done that in our office, never to resume the smoking. If your power of will is not strong enough now, begin to build it up, till some fine morning you can say to yourself that tobacco is no longer your master. The best way to stop is to stop.

"At this point we suppose a thousand women or more have told us, 'But, doctor, that is easy to say and hard to do.' Well, maybe so, but you are a human being and you have a backbone. Besides, you are starting with a disease that cripples more human beings than any other disease. Do you desire health, or are you going to take the chance on chronic arthritis and crippling? Yours is the choice.

"You say that you have been drinking very little water, maybe only one or two glasses a day, and not more than three. Water is the only compound that has the ability to carry or float the poisonous waste from the body cells to the four great eliminating organs—and these poisonous wastes or toxic materials are the very things that make you ill; they are the compounds that build up the autointoxication that is back of arthritis. The practical application of this scientific fact is to drink at least five glasses of water every day—and when we say water we mean water; no, we do not mean soup or juice or milk or coffee or tea or broth—we mean water.

"And your food intake has been such that it has acidulated your body—cereals, breadstuffs, eggs, meats and most of the 'made' desserts add to the body acidity—they are acidulating foods. Instead of taking a breakfast of cereal, toast with butter and coffee, which is a completely acidulating meal that makes arthritis worse, take an alkalizing meal of nothing but fruits until your hands clear up, until you get most of the stored poisons out of your body, say,

A BREAKFAST OF

Orange juice or half a mild grapefruit
Either sweet pears or sweet grapes
Ripe banana either raw or baked
Take or omit four ounces of milk

"Please note that this breakfast is totally alkalizing, that it helps to overcome the toxic acidity that is the basis of arthritis.

"You say that your lunch has usually been a meat soup, a meat sandwich, and cake or cookies, with a cup of coffee—seldom any vegetables or fruits. Such a meal is almost totally acidulating. We suggest that you substitute a meal on the alkalizing side. Yes, we know about the high-protein trend that has been in the mind of the public and the profession for some time, but our experience says it is a mistake, so we shall plan so there will be no meat in

THE LUNCH

Six ounces of vegetable juice
With a dash of lemon juice
A large dish of green (young) lima beans
Toasted yellow corn muffins with butter
A dish of raspberries with cream

"The vegetable juice, the lima beans and the raspberries are alkalizing, preventing any acidulation of the body by the corn muffins. Simple, but very scientific!

"Your dinners have been fair, but you should avoid all soups with meat stock or meat. You should also avoid beef and pork in every form, including ham and bacon, until the arthritic poisons are overcome. And you should use only the meats from rather young animals and birds, as well as fish from the ocean seas (as Columbus expressed it) or eggs. Your desserts should be melons, or berries or other fruits. Please remember that you are not to eat such devitalized foods as white sugar or white flour, or any of the foods that contain them—no white breadstuffs, or cakes, or cookies or pie crusts or other pastries. Bearing these things in mind, let us make up for you a

WHOLESOME DINNER

Tender lettuce, tomato slices, avocado strips
Swiss chard   Fresh green peas
Potatoes, either cooked in jacket or baked
Boiled scrod (or baked), with lemon quarters
Cantaloupes or sliced peaches

"This whole meal is alkalizing except the scrod. Yes, potatoes when baked or cooked in the jacket are alkalizing, as is the rest of the meal, so it helps to overcome the arthritis. Use salt in moderation but no strong condiments or sauces or spices, such as pepper; if you wish the mild paprika, there is no objection. If summer has been in mind in making up this plan, it does not matter, for in winter use the vegetables and fruits available at this season; for instance, baked Rome beauty apples in place of cantaloupes and cherries; grapes or sweet pears in place of berries.

"You say you are in the open air very little. Walk in the open on beautiful days and freely help yourself to fresh air—be thankful that your feet and legs have not shown rheumatic or arthritic tendencies. And you also say that the intestines do not always work so well. That makes it important for you to go to the bathroom soon after breakfast, also soon after dinner, and solicit an action; cultivate the habit of regularity of bowel function, and maintain that regularity for life by obeying the calls of Nature."

All who tend towards constipation should read the chapter on the subject in this book.

And now you have the record of what we have told our patients, mostly women, for decades. Of course, we have written out the instructions for them. Please note the simplicity of these recommendations. We repeat, those women who cooperated with us have always cleared up, without exception.

LIVE THESE TEACHINGS FOR RESULTS

Often we reminded them that merely reading their instructions would not help them; they had to practice the knowledge we gave them, live this knowledge, to get results. And so it is with this book: If you have rheumatism or arthritis, you have to live these teachings to get results. Let us illustrate:

A young woman from Canada—in her late thirties—developed the acute rheumatoid arthritis we have here discussed. She had remissions between the attacks, so she made up her mind she was well —until the next attack occurred. Each attack was a little worse, and lasted a little longer. We pleaded with her that correct living habits were a small and easy price to pay to ward off crippling arthritis. She did not heed, but told us later that she passed off the warnings with the attitude that doctors are alarmists. So after she had had quite a few attacks of the acute arthritis, the disease took possession, and did not leave.

Years later she was brought to us on a stretcher, unable to use either arms or legs, and full of pain. She wept when she saw us and said, "If I had only heeded your advice years ago!" On making the examination we found that some of her joints were limed up—ankylosed—while some were rigid because of the pain. We had to tell her that the joints that were physiologically ankylosed were lost for good; that with careful living she could become painfree, and regain much motion in the joints held fixed by pain. In other words, she would be partly crippled for life but she could gain ease of body and mobility of some of the joints that were rigid.

It was a tragic penalty to pay for not accepting and heeding the truth when it could and would have made her whole and well. "The truth shall set you free," but it has to be lived to accomplish this.

It was different with Bob. He was only seventeen years old, but he wanted health. His parents had been too busy making a success in their shop to give time enough to his raising and his education; they needed him as a helper to make the shop even more successful, so his schooling had stopped. The

mother did not have time to prepare regular meals,
so they lived on bread and coffee; on cheese, bread
and coffee; on meat, bread, pie and coffee—yes,
these were the meals. The boy became toxic and
developed acute rheumatoid arthritis, with painful, stiff, swollen fingers. We instructed him how
to live, and emphasized the consumption of
fruits, vegetables and water always thereafter, so
he would remain well. Five weeks after he
started the good care, his hands felt and looked
normal; in ordinary usage there was no more pain
—it took very heavy pressure to bring out any discomfort. He went on to good health and remained
well as long as we contacted him. His parents were
too busy to come with him even once; they were
even too busy to send word that they appreciated
his recovery. But Bob was a fine boy.

The reasons for such a quick recovery were his
youth, also his following directions to the letter—
yes, a fine boy.

Still different was the lady of twenty-six. The
first month under our care she lost every bad symp-
tom of arthritis—soreness, stiffness, swelling and
disability—she was in the early stages of the disease. We asked her to stay under observation till
she recovered, explaining that although the symptoms had vanished, she was still toxic, for which
reason the arthritis could, and almost surely would
return, if correct care were lacking. But no, she felt
well and was youthfully certain that health was

hers, so she was going to do as she pleased. She did. About six months later she requested reinstatement as a patient. "I have learned my lesson," she said. "This time I am going to recover and stay well." And she did.

The moral of these tales is that those who learn the truth and live it recover from acute arthritis.

10 Feeding in Arthritis

The first rule in feeding any sick person is to select wholesome foods and prepare them so as to retain their health value.

The second rule is to eat slowly and masticate well at every meal. There are no teeth in the intestines. The stomach is a receptacle for foods and drinks, but only a little digesting takes place there; the small intestines are the main laboratories in which the food is digested, that is, prepared to become blood.

But rules and teachings are worthless unless they are used. A patient who has read many of our writings remarked the other day, "I have read much but practiced little of your teachings—that is why I am ill and have to consult you." How true!

So please remember that merely reading this book on rheumatism and arthritis will not clear up any disease; you have to live these teachings, these truths, to obtain the benefits. Thousands have lived them and recovered from rheumatism and arthritis.

The fact that white sugar and white flour are de-vitalized foods has been explained in another chapter; they should not be eaten. The evils of frying have also been explained—please dispense with the frying pan, and do no greasy cooking; use no thickened gravies or sauces of any kind, and no stuffings (or dressings) in preparing meat or fish. Please study with care the chapter on Food and Cooking.

There is much propaganda to the effect that it is necessary to eat a heavy breakfast, and it is natural for those who process and sell special foods eaten in this meal to desire to dispose of as much of them as possible. But the truth is that arthritics should eat a moderate breakfast—as much food as the body needs, but no more. We are told that the body has gone without food for a long time—since the dinner of the previous day—and hence much food is needed for breakfast? But what does the body do between dinner and breakfast? Generally the life is very easy and most of the hours are spent in sleep so there is no need of cereal with sugar and cream, ham or bacon with eggs, toast with butter and jam, and coffee with sugar and cream. Meals like this fill the body with more acid, and help to build disease, including rheumatism and arthritis.

When we encounter a person suffering with arthritis, we have the problem of ridding his body of stored toxicity (acid wastes) and restoring the normal tone and health of the body, including the mildly alkaline or neutral reaction that exists in health. We do this in part through the feeding, which is one of the most important health measures in this disease.

BEST FOODS FOR ARTHRITICS

The most important health foods in arthritis and rheumatism are the fresh vegetables, which should be eaten in generous amounts both for lunch and for dinner.

The second most important health foods are the fresh fruits, which should make up a large part of the breakfast; they should also be used as dessert, to the exclusion of cakes, cookies, pies and puddings.

And the patient should get away from heavy sweetening of foods and drinks—no white sugar, please remember. If sweetening is desired, use honey, or brown sugar (which is exactly the same thing as raw sugar), maple sugar or syrup. Or eat seedless raisins, dates, figs or sweet prunes, all of which winter fruits are stuffed full of Nature's own vital sugar—dates may be more than 70% natural sugar. Molasses taken early in the sugar-making process is quite good, but the blackstrap molasses has been cooked to death and is a rather inferior product. The Department of Agriculture has said it is only fit for cattle food, but some men and women consume it because they have read that it is a superior product, which it is not. The sugars and sweets we have discussed in this paragraph are Nature's own sweets and they are good, but they should be taken in moderation.

WARNING ON FOOD ACIDS

One fact about rheumatism and arthritis must be stressed. Those who are in this toxic state become sensitive to food acids, no matter how good they may be—the chief of these acids are citric, malic and tartaric. For this reason many of these patients have to take the highly acid fruits, such as lemon, limes, oranges and grapefruit in moderation. The milder apples like Macintosh, Rome beauty and delicious they may eat, but very tart apples are better omitted; sweet pears, sweet grapes, and mild peaches and apricots are fine, and so are ripe bananas—no green showing on the peel at the tip. So please remember that many arthritics should not have more than one glass of fruit juice per day, and should avoid the very tart or sour fruits, but take the mild fruits instead. When a person becomes sensitive to food acids, he grows sorer and more painful if he takes much of them.

It is customary to eat breakfast cereals. We have

nothing whatever against these foods, as foods, if
they are made of the whole grain. But nobody eats
them slowly and chews them well, so as to start the
digestion right—the first part of starch digestion
should take place in the mouth, for the saliva contains a digestive ferment, ptyalin, which begins to
turn the starch into a form of sugar—that is one reason we should eat slowly and chew well. However,
cereals are swallowed so fast and masticated so little that the ptyalin action is aborted—which easily
leads to some indigestion with excessive gas and
inferior blood, and this makes up a disease tendency.

So we instruct our patients to take whole wheat
toast, which they have to chew, for we also add, no
drinking of any fluid during any meal. Take beverages or other fluids at the beginning or the end of
meals, and water may be drunk between meals as
often as desired. But foods should not be washed
down with liquids.

HEALTH BUILDING BREAKFASTS

The breakfast should be moderate in amount and
a simple meal. The truth is that moderation in eating is a cornerstone of health. The majority in our
land overeat. Rheumatics and arthritics should
eat enough, but no more, at any meal; they should

never eat until they have that full feeling; they should always leave the table with the feeling that they could comfortably eat some more.

The old Greeks had a motto, nothing to excess; this is moderation in all things, which should be the motto of every arthritic at every meal.

It is usual, but not necessary, to eat some starch in every breakfast, usually a cereal, or toast; or cereal and toast, which leads to overeating of starch and execessive body acidity.

We need no breakfast starch, especially when recovering from disease, for we have some sugary fruits that serve even better: They are raisins, figs, dates, and sweet prunes (not the tart prunes), and thoroughly ripe bananas—green bananas are about as starchy as white potatoes, but ripe bananas contain almost no starch for nearly all of it turns to sugar in the ripening process.

Let us plan some breakfasts for the benefit of rheumatic and arthritic individuals who desire to live so as to rebuild their health:

BREAKFASTS

Orange juice
Unsweetened apple sauce
Seedless raisins
An ounce or less pecan meats

Grapefruit or grapefruit juice
Sweet pears
Thoroughly ripe bananas

Tomato juice, no salt, no spicing
Peaches
Figs and nothing more

Large serving of cantaloupe
Apricots or baked apple
Stewed sweet prunes—no sugar added
A few almonds, if desired

A large orange or orange juice
Cherries
Stewed figs
A glass of milk

Honeydew melon
Unsugared apple sauce with cottage cheese
Ripe bananas, cooked or raw

Yes, these are simple, but nourishing meals.
Weight for weight, raisins, figs, dates and sweet
prunes are more nourishing than toast and far more
nourishing than bread, while ripe bananas are
about as nourishing as white potatoes.

You will notice that we have permitted nut
meats, or milk, or cottage cheese with these fruit
breakfasts—only one of these should be taken in a

breakfast; for instance, if a glass of milk is taken then there will be no cheese or nuts in the meal.

So you may make your own fruit breakfast menus that are both wholesome and nourishing, please note: The breakfast begins with either fruit juice, or else a citrus fruit like orange or grapefruit, or melon; second, we have another ordinary fruit found in the market, such as apples, pears, peaches, apricots or cherries; third, we select one of the highly nourishing or sugary fruits, such as raisins, figs, dates, sweet prunes, or ripe bananas; fourth, we either add or omit, a few nut meats, or a glass of milk, or an order of cottage cheese, not more than three or four ounces of the latter.

Such a breakfast is tasty, health-building and nourishing.

But what about a beverage? That usually means coffee, tea, chocolate or cocoa. All of these contain the poison caffeine, under three names—theine, theobromine and caffeine—all identical, all toxic to the human body, all with a tendency to make disease, including arthritis, worse. So what are you to do? It is best not to take any of these while trying to rid the body of disease—and at all other times. But if you are in earnest, you can at least cut the coffee consumption down to one cup of unsweetened coffee per day, and omit the other three drinks—cocoa, chocolate and tea.

While we think that fruit breakfasts are best, we also know that human beings are human, and some

will not go the full distance. So let us give some
breakfast menus containing one starch, but when
we add the starch, please note, we do not add any
milk or cheese or nuts. If you are in earnest about
ridding the body of arthritis, the breakfast has to
be simple.

FRUIT BREAKFASTS WITH STARCH

If the digestion is faulty, take the fruit juice about
thirty or forty minutes before eating the solid part
of the breakfast.

And please remember that with toast or muffins
or sticks, butter or good margarine is permitted as
dressing.

When there is starch in the breakfast, omit the
nut meats, the cottage cheese; take milk seldom in
such breakfasts. It is important to eat in moderation and too great variety can easily lead to overeating.

Also remember that all starches require extra
good mastication.

FRUIT AND STARCH BREAKFASTS

Orange juice (30 mins. before the solid food)
Sweet grapes
Toasted bread with butter
Beverage at the end of the meal

Grapefruit, or grapefruit juice
Ripe bananas
Yellow corn sticks with butter
Beverage at the end of the meal

Unsweetened pineapple juice
Baked apple, no sugar added
Whole wheat raisin muffins, butter
Beverage at the end of the meal

Honeydew melon
Sweet pears
Yellow corn muffins with butter
Beverage at the end of the meal

Sliced oranges flecked with date meats
Unsweetened apple sauce
Whole wheat raisin toast with butter
A glass of milk

"Beverage at the end of the meal" has been repeated on purpose, to remind you that you are not to drink during the meal, for such drinking in the end results in too limited mastication.

But what kind of beverages are you to take? We hope it is not coffee or tea—or at least that it will not be more than one cup a day of either coffee or tea, for these two drinks add to the body toxicity, and hence to the disease; the same is true of chocolate and cocoa, which should be omitted.

Some like mint tea; others are partial to alfalfa tea; and there are various non-toxic beverages on the market referred to as cereal drinks; those who love coffee too much may take Sanka, which is real coffee with nearly all of the poison removed. God gave us the best of all beverages, water; how we would treasure it if we had to pay from fifteen cents to a dollar for a little glass at a bar!! Water may be taken hot or cool; if the digestion is troublesome, hot water is best near mealtimes. Ice water should be avoided for it interferes with good digestion.

LUNCHES

You will notice that the purpose of the breakfasts has been to make them refreshing, that is, of such a nature that they build health, at the same time giving enough food to nourish the body. We have heard much talk about having plenty of protein in the meals, so we must call your attention to the fact that an excessive amount of protein makes the arthritis worse—to clear up rheumatic ills it is necessary to take protein in moderation. We have not featured protein in the breakfasts, nor shall we do so in the lunches. And here we wish to call something very important to your attention:

While clearing up rheumatism or arthritis, do not take protein more than once or twice per day.

If you wish protein in the lunch, do not take it in the breakfast; if you have it in the breakfast, then take no protein in the lunch. Repetition, take protein only once or twice a day. (Milk, cheese, eggs, fish and meat are proteins; although nut meats are chiefly fatty foods, for the purpose of arthritic recovery, we have to put nuts among the proteins.)

The only meal in which a full protein portion is to be eaten is the dinner. As fruits are the backbone of the breakfast, so vegetables are the foundation of the lunch. Here is another important fact to bear in mind: Vegetables are the most important of all foods in overcoming rheumatism and arthritis, and the vegetables are to be both cooked and raw.

RAW VS. COOKED VEGETABLES

At this point so many with a little dietetic knowledge go wrong: They have heard that the raw vegetables are better than the cooked ones, being more vital. They are more vital, but in the long run they are not better. The raw vegetables are rich in minerals and vitamins and chlorophyll, and the ones that are green in color have the most vital value. But the raw vegetables are also heavily endowed with hard cellulose, which is upsetting to the digestion of many who lack full digestive power; then the large amount of cellulose strongly tends to create much internal gas, which is one evidence of indigestion.

Cooking breaks down the cellulose so it does not interfere much with the digestion. We have been consulted by whole families who had been converted to the raw vegetable, or rather, raw diet idea. Theoretically that is fine. Practically, it made of them perambulating gas factories. The best policy is to balance up matters and take some of the vegetables raw and some of them cooked, and this is how we shall manage matters in making the menus.

LUNCHES FOR ARTHRITICS

Celery hearts and radishes
Broccoli cooked with the tender little leaves
Whole wheat raisin bread, butter
Baked apple stuffed with well soaked raisins

How is one to dress wholesome meals so they remain in the health-building class? First of all, in moderation. A meal of this kind could be so overloaded with butter, oil and cream that it would lead to overeating, for all of these dressings are fat concentrations. So please remember that dressings are to be used rather sparingly. With the celery and radishes one may have salt in moderation, some lemon juice and a little oil, or a little mayonnaise

dressing; the broccoli may be moderately salted
while cooking—never use large quantities of salt;
the butter on the bread should be a moderate
amount, not above average; the same is true of the
apple, if cream should be used. Fruits are so delicious that they do not need the cream, but it is
permitted occasionally for the sake of variety. As
for sweetening of fruits. Why? These excellent
foods have a fine flavor of their own. No white
sugar at any time, please. Honey or maple sugar
(or maple syrup) or brown sugar (which is often
called raw sugar) are the best dressings if sweeteners are desired. Use them too in moderation.

As for the powerful spices and sauces, avoid
them for they irritate the digestive organs. When
people had no refrigeration, and had to use high
seasoning to preserve foods and to hide the bad
odors of foods that were already beginning to spoil,
there may have been some justification for dousing
them with pepper, mustard and horseradish; with
our refrigeration there is no excuse for that kind
of seasoning. Avoid strong and heavy seasoning,
for the sake of your health.

As for acid dressing, lemon juice is superior to
vinegar.

French endive with mayonnaise
Baby carrots and peas with
Little spring potatoes
Black Mission figs.

Head lettuce with oil and lemon juice
Stewed scallions with butter
Yellow corn muffins
A few nut meats

Diced fresh pineapple on
Lettuce leaves with cottage cheese
Baked egg plant, large serving
Whole wheat bread sticks, butter
Sweet grapes

Cucumber slices with avocado and lemon juice
Cooked green lima beans
Whole wheat raisin muffins
Sweet pear, raw or baked

Diced raw apple and seedless raisins on
Lettuce leaves, dotted with whipped cream
Cooked summer squash, large serving
Whole wheat Melba toast
Glass of milk, if desired, at end of meal

Radishes, carrot sticks and ripe olives
Cooked green peas, with real cream
Whole rice with raisins, butter sauce
Grapes and a few nuts

As the vegetables are so important, it is essential to prepare them right. The raw vegetables present very little difficulty, for they need only to be

well washed; of course, it is a good idea to present
them attractively, and then there is the question of
dressing. Most of them have such fine flavor that
our favorite dressing is no dressing at all. However, such simple tastes do not generally prevail.
The best acid is lemon or lime juice, or other raw
fruit juice; with this may be used any edible oil,
such as olive, peanut oil, soy oil, corn oil. Sometimes mayonnaise may be used. If the salad contains fruit, a tasty dressing may be whipped cream,
or cottage cheese—cottage cheese goes well with
vegetable salads too. Salt in moderation is permitted. When one uses ripe tomatoes and avocado
strips, no other dressing is essential, for the tomato
gives the acidity and the avocado furnishes the
oil. A little salt may be added.

BASIC RECIPE FOR COOKING VEGETABLES

The basic recipe for cooking vegetables is very
simple: Wash the vegetables and if necessary cut
them into pieces and cook in so little water that
there is none to throw away. Eat or drink your
share of the cooking liquor. A little salt may be
added to the cooking water. Never cook vegetables
with fat or meat, for that makes them difficult to
digest. Vegetables may be plainly cooked, or

steamed, or pressure cooked, or cooked in Dutch oven, but always conserve the cooking liquor; some vegetables may be baked. Never fry the vegetables. Leafy vegetables, like spinach, cook in the water adhering to the leaves and their own juices. Open kettle cooking destroys more vitamins than any other method; pressure cooking preserves most of the vitamins, for most of the oxygen is exhausted before the cooking process begins, and the cooking is done in such a short time. It is not the heat that is chiefly at fault in destroying vitamins. It is the oxidation.

We hear that in arthritis tomatoes and spinach and other vegetables should not be eaten because "they contain oxalic acid." It is true that some vegetables contain oxalic acid, but it is so little that it does no harm. Spinach, for instance, contains a trace of oxalic acid, but it is so little that if you were to eat a bushel of it, no harm would be done. Tomatoes are good, but due to their acidity they should be eaten in moderation in arthritis, especially if tenderness, soreness or pain are present; tomatoes should be red ripe all over for arthritics, not green in color.

There is only one common vegetable that contains so much oxalic acid that it should be avoided; this is rhubarb; it is objectionable not only on account of its oxalic acid, but because it is dressed with large amounts of white sugar.

These statements are based on scientific research by careful scientists. So enjoy your spinach, turnip tops, beet tops, chard and other leafy greens, for they are rich in organic mineral salts, including calcium; also in vitamins and chlorophyll—they are very desirable vegetables in arthritis—yes, both in health and disease.

DINNER MENUS

In the dinners, raw and cooked vegetables play the most important part in restoring health. So we have a good raw salad, and plenty of cooked vegetables.

Fruit we use as dessert, for it helps the vegetables in building health.

The protein is the most controversial ingredient in the dinner, so we shall explain about various proteins. The majority like meat or fish best, so here is some information for meat and fish eaters. The best fish comes from the ocean, for it is so rich in organic mineral salts and vitamins—fresh-water fish is not so well endowed. Pork is too rich, too fatty, as a protein in arthritis, and as it is force fed in it contains too much waste for a sick person. Beef is also force fed, so it should be used seldom. The best meats for sick persons are the young meats, such as chicken, turkey, veal, lamb, and fish from the ocean.

Cheese, especially cottage cheese, milk and eggs may be selected as dinner proteins. But there is one point to remember: Take only one protein in each dinner; for instance, if fish is the protein, do not eat eggs, or milk or meat in the same meal.

Those who are fond of legumes and digest them well may take lentils, or dried peas, or dried beans as the dinner protein.

Some believe they can get their protein from the avocado, but this is not true, for the avocado is a fatty fruit, with very little protein, two percent or less. Use the avocado as fatty dressing on fruits and vegetables. Likewise, nuts are not satisfactory proteins, for they are primarily fatty or oily foods, some of them containing a goodly amount of protein; but to obtain enough of the protein, one has to overeat of the nut oil, and that is bad from the health standpoint. The remarks about dressing foods for lunch also hold for the dinners.

A final reminder: Avoid all frying; have no thickened gravies or sauces on any foods, and use no starchy stuffings or dressings with meat or fish—if you feel the need of such dressing, make it of vegetables.

DINNERS FOR ARTHRITICS

Celery, ripe olives and carrot sticks
Swiss chard   Stewed onions

Roast lamb   Mint flavored unsweetened apple
   sauce
Baked potato (if hungry for it)
Sweet grapes for dessert

Lettuce and tomato salad with radishes
Carrots   Spinach
Roast chicken with unthickened giblet sauce
Cooked small spring potatoes
Baked banana with shredded coconut

Cucumber slices and ripe olives
String beans   Green lima beans
Baked or broiled fish, parsley and lemon
Jacket-cooked potatoes
Sliced ripe peaches

Head lettuce with orange sections
Beet tops   Green peas
Roast turkey with unsweetened apple sauce
Yams, cooked in the jacket
A dish of sweet cherries

French endive, grated carrots
Broccoli   Lima beans
Omelette with fine-cut green pepper
Baked sweet potato
Ripe apricots   Cream

Large salad of lettuce, chopped raw
      apple and orange sections, with full
      portion of cottage cheese
Large dish of green peas
Baked apple with cream

Please remember, there is to be no bread, no
flour product, in the dinner. That is final, if you
wish the best results. Hundreds of arthritics have
told me, "I thought you meant me to have bread if
I left out the potatoes." No bread in the dinner at
any time, please.

As for potatoes, they are permitted, if baked or
jacket-cooked, for then they are alkalizing—the
bread is acidulating. If hungry enough to need
starch in the dinner, let the starch be white potato,
or sweet potato, or yam. If not hungry, leave the
potato out.

Soup, though popular, is best omitted, except
vegetable soup, with no meat or meat stock in it.

Meals like these, if slowly eaten and well masticated, help to alkalize and purify the body, and
thus they help overcome rheumatic and arthritic
disease. But remember, eating is not all there is to
recovery. Right drinking, right cleansing, and right
thinking are just as important.

When we speak of meat, it means the flesh of animals, birds and fish—yes, chicken and turkey and
fish are meats, from the dietetic standpoint.

There is no hardship in correct eating for the sake of building health, for the foods are the best obtainable, the finest, most delicious products of the land and sea.

11 Treatments

SUNSHINE   AIR   WATER
EXERCISE   RAYS   MEDICATION

For more than forty years we have seen treatments and cures of arthritis come and go; the only thing we have found effective in all of these years has been the remedial way of correct living that we outline in this book.

The most dramatic cures that have excited the public during this time were the cortisone and ACTH that were hailed by many as the true solution to this ancient ailment. When these remedies first appeared they were expensive, for they had to be extracted from little glands adjacent to the kidneys, or from another gland at the base of the brain. We heard people bemoaning the fact that they were unable to pay $20.00 a dose for these wonderful cures!

But what happened? There were wonderful remissions, and the fortunate ones thought they were making speedy recoveries. But unfortunately, the patients could not continue taking these hormones; they were too powerful. They upset the body and even changed the shape of the face. And when the patients stopped taking the remedies the arthritis returned. Some deaths were reported to us by the families, stating that either cortisone or ACTH destroyed life. Now the public is not relying on these two hormones to overcome arthritis.

If you will only think the thing through, you will realize that a disease caused by wrong living—such as deficient water drinking, injudicious eating, constipation, insufficient exercise and the resultant toxicity—can not be expected to clear up by taking some doses of poisonous medicine; and you will further realize that the logical and true conquest of such a disease is by removing the cause of the disease—wrong living—and substituting correct, hygienic living.

SUNSHINE

Sunlight is the source of all animate life on this planet. With moisture and carbonic acid gas, the rays of the sun developed vegetation until it was able to support a higher type of life, animal life. And this must have continued for eons before man

could appear on the scene, fragile man who has to
be coddled in the right temperature, in an atmos-
phere rich in oxygen, from sea level to a few thousand feet of elevation. If man is deprived of air, he
can live only a few minutes; if deprived of water,
he can live but a few days; if deprived of food, only
about a month—if he is fat he can live two months
or longer, with good care.

Sunlight also helps to sustain health. An occasional person is allergic to sunshine, and compelled
to live in the shade to remain comfortable. But
nearly all flourish with their quota of sunshine.
Those who are much housed should make a point
of walking or living in the sun whenever possible.
But they should avoid overexposure, for excessive
exposure may produce serious disease. All know
about heatstroke and sunstroke, which may disable
a person for months, or even destroy life. Excessive
sunshine, especially when the weather is very hot,
may so adversely affect the blood corpuscles that
life is lost.

Those with heavily pigmented skin tolerate the
sun better than those who are fair. The general
rule is not to stay in the sun all day when it is very
hot, especially not in the midday sun; this is most
important for those who are blond. If it is necessary to be in the sun all day at such times, cover
the head, but have the covering ventilated, and it
is well to have a piece of cloth wrung out of water
inside of the hat or cap. Even so, take advantage

of shade when present, and wear light garments, light in both weight and color.

Those who are unable to spend much time in the sun may obtain the same results by taking sun-baths, either in the nude or wearing a minimum amount of clothing. If not accustomed to the sun, begin with not more than five minutes on each of the four body surfaces—front, back and two sides. That means, not more than twenty minutes of sun-bathing the first day; if fair of skin, increase one minute each day until each body surface receives fifteen minutes of sunshine—a total of one hour for the nude or near-nude sunbath; if dark of skin, the increase of time may be more rapid, and the length of the sunbath may be about an hour and twenty minutes. This is playing safe. Sunshine and sun-baths are good in arthritis.

But avoid overly long sunbaths, and never, never, never fall asleep in the hot sun, for the re-sulting burn may be severe to the point of great danger, and the healing process is tedious.

Those who are unable to take advantage of real sunshine may use the sun lamp. As each lamp has its own strength, it is important to learn how long it is to be used on each body surface. Begin with a short application of the lamp, and gradually in-crease to the point of normal dosage. Always pro-tect the eyes from strong sun lamp rays by wearing dark glasses.

Please do not expect sunshine or sun lamps to

cure; their function is to aid in toning and vitaliz-ing the body.

FRESH AIR

Clean, fresh air is important, for it is a basic ingre-dient of the blood; it contains the oxygen, in the best form, needed by the blood stream for all parts of the body; the oxygen unites with the hemo-globin of the red blood corpuscles and forms oxy-hemoglobin, and so it is carried to every nook and corner of the body; all the tissues help themselves to what oxygen they need; in the tissues, and espe-cially in the muscles, the oxygen supports the combustion that burns the wastage of the body, so it can be cast out of the system. This waste is car-ried away again by the blood, in such forms as carbonic acid gas, which leaves by way of the lungs—if this could be consolidated it would form several ounces of carbon or coal each day; or as urea and its modifications or as uric acid in various forms which urates are carried to the kidneys and there separated from the blood to be excreted in the urine; or as other acids that leave by way of the skin; or by way of the great sewer of the body, the colon. It is the oxygen of the air that supports the combustion within the body that enables the sys-tem to rid itself of its poisonous wastes; and it is the blood that carts away the toxic waste so it can be excreted by the four great eliminating systems of the body—the skin, the lungs, the kidneys and the large intestine.

Combustion within the body! At first this might seem odd, but it is the slow fire of life that has to keep burning, for when it is extinguished it means physical death.

And all these wastes are poisonous to the body that produces them. This means that if they are retained within the body, they intoxicate the system and make it ill. When you realize this, do you wonder that we tell you not to tolerate constipation? That we say, breathe fresh air? That we ask you to tone up your body with exercises, if you are to take them, and let the sun shine on you as a tonic to the body, more especially the skin? Did you realize that sunshine contacting the skin creates vitamin D, a precious substance needed to maintain health?

And please remember that when the wastes produced in the living process are retained, in perceptible degree, the body becomes more and more toxic, which is autointoxication or toxemia; and furthermore, this is the basis of chronic diseases.

The air is free. Help yourself to it day and night. If you are housed in your work, do your best to have ventilation; if you work where the air is filthy, as it is in many large cities, and industrial districts, then try to live where the air is good. At night ventilate well, but it is not good for arthritics to be in draughts, for they tend to produce congestion.

Place the bed so there is ventilation without draught; one may also use screens.

How about deep breathing? A few deep breaths while taking a good straight posture are fine. But to do extensive deep breathing gets no more oxygen into the tissues, for the body uses oxygen according to activity. To be sure to use more oxygen, one has to do more physical work or exercise. But good posture is always helpful, and to spend time in the pure fresh air aids in building and maintaining health. Walking is one of the best of tonics.

But in arthritis walks and exercises may have to be restricted; however good ventilation and plenty of fresh air are valuable self-treatments.

WATER, INTERNALLY AND EXTERNALLY

Elsewhere we have laid down the rule that a small person should drink at least five glasses of water daily, and a large one about eight glasses of water per day—we refer to a glass as eight ounces of water. A rough modification of this rule is: Drink a glass (eight ounces) of water daily for each twenty pounds of body weight.

When we say water, we mean water. Thousands of times our patients have interpreted water to mean tea, coffee, chocolate, milk, soup or juice. Wrong interpretation! We mean water. In the same way, when we have told catarrhal patients not to eat cheese of any kind, hundreds of them have responded, "But that does not mean cottage cheese." But it does. Life is fun, and often funny.

Please drink your share of water every day, for there is no other substance that will float the disease-producing poisons out of the body. We regret that a few men who should have known better broadcast the idea "to drink only when thirsty." The fact is that we need water daily whether thirsty or not, whether the weather is hot or cold and when we do not drink enough water our bodies become toxic, that is, diseased. In arthritis there is a special reason for drinking water—the body is already diseased and needs to rid itself of stored poisonous wastes.

The regular bath, if the patient is able to enter and leave the tub, may be used as an aid. Fill the tub with comfortably hot water and submerge every afflicted joint in the bath water and soak in it for about fifteen minutes, or a little longer, if the body is vigorous; if the body is sensitive, for a shorter time. Do not continue the hot soaking until exhaustion sets in. After the hot bath is the best time for straightening the limbs and for moderate exercising of said limbs, if the joints are badly afflicted.

Steam baths, or cabinet baths serve the same purpose as the hot bath; again, do not continue them until exhaustion sets in.

Those who are unable to use the tub may use
the hot pack, which is best given as follows: Tear
up some worn linen, like old sneets or pillowslips,
so that when folded four-ply (four thickness of
cloth) the piece of cloth to be used covers the
painful joint. Dip four-ply cloth in water as not
as the hands can bear, wring out so the cloth does
not drip, and apply four-ply at once over the bad
joint; immediately cover the wet cloth with soft,
dry woollen; fix in place and leave on for an hour.
This may be used once or more each day.

Badly afflicted hands and wrists may be soaked
in a basin of hot water for fifteen or twenty minutes.

Epsom salts may or may not be added to soaking
water, in bathtub or basin, as desired.

In arthritis it is best to avoid cold applications
and cold baths.

Arthritics who take Turkish baths should avoid
the cold plunge.

In the past many of our patients have been told
how to use the hot wet pack, and they have used
a regular washcloth to wring out of hot water, and
a dry turkish towel to cover the wet cloth. That is
one way of following directions, but not the right
way. No oil cloths, no rubber sheets in the not wet
pack, please.

And please remember that the best and most

important water treatment is to drink from five to eight glasses of water daily, according to body weight.

EXERCISE IN ARTHRITIS

If the upper part of the body is afflicted, and the legs and feet are all right, then walk and take moderate exercises for the legs—but no violent exercises.

If the legs and feet are afflicted, and the arms and hands are all right, then take moderate exercises for the arms and shoulders, but no violent movements, please.

If only the spine is arthritic, exercise the rest of the body, but avoid exercises that compel forceful movement of the spine.

In other words, the affected, afflicted joints are to be exercised in moderation. No forceful, violent movements, please, no prolonged and hard work for them, for heavy exercises make conditions worse.

One patient had finally become comfortable again, after years of pains in hips, knees and ankles. He formerly loved to climb a steep hill near his home. So we warned him that this was a danger point in his progress (the danger is tendency to overdo at this stage) and for this reason he must avoid overusing of the legs; take only short walks on the level—no up-hill or down-hill walking; no

standing for a long time. Just be moderate in all
things.

All of these things we told him with emphasis.
But he felt so good that he climbed the steep hill
once, and then he descended; and still he felt fine,
so up and down he went once more. He triumph-
antly telephoned us what he had done, adding that
it did not hurt him one bit, that all was just fine.
He felt hurt when we answered, "Wait until to-
morrow. Benjamin Franklin said, 'Experience
keeps a dear school, but fools will learn in no
other.'"

It required over a month of good care to overcome the damage he did himself on that hillside,
and to get rid of the pain once more. He recovered
so he could climb all the hills he wished to conquer as often as he desired, by being careful.

What kind of exercises? Avoid the short, choppy
and violent exercises. Take the large and sweep-
ing exercises; for the upper part of the body use
calisthenics for the arms, rotating movements for
the shoulders and the neck, but not choppy and
never violent. For the spine, bend backward and
forward with firm, steady turning or twisting at
the waist, rotating the body from side to side; for
the abdomen and legs, the repeated squat, but not
jerkily—the squat is also known as the deep-knee
bend; for the legs, walking and the supine exercises with legs in the air, going through the movement of riding the bicycle, or else hold the legs as

straight in the knee region as possible and alter-
nately raise the legs; after getting expert, raise
both legs, held as straight at the knee as possible.
These are the basic suggestions to which one may
add many modifications.

But never overdo the exercising of the affected
parts. One can only do harm with much exercise
for the afflicted joints, for excessive exercise in-
jures the joints, makes the disease worse, and pro-
longs the recovery. There are times when rest is
more important than exercise.

But always do your best to maintain the full mobility of the joints; the best time to stretch the
joints is after the hot bath.

RAYS OR RADIATION

Various rays are helpful in the healing art; the
X-Ray has aided us in finding out the truth about
internal conditions, playing an important part in
surgery; the infra-red is a penetrating and warming
ray that often brings ease and relief in deep seated
pains; the sun lamp gives artificial sunshine when
the real article is not available, and it is easy to
control as to length and strength of treatments,
but it does not fully take the place of sunshine.
For instance, real sunshine is helpful in clearing up
the lesions of psoriasis—we have seen no such results with sun lamps.

X-Rays should not be used by amateurs; even professionals overuse them too often. When overused they irritate—years ago many of those who used them developed cancers of the body parts much exposed to them, especially the fingers and hands.

We doubt the advisability of turning violet rays over to amateurs; it is easy to overapply them.

Sun lamps (the mercury-quartz are considered the best, but reliable electric companies put out some good ones too) and infra-red lamps may be used by careful, responsible lay persons. Of course, they should carefully find out about dosages, which differ with the strength of the lamps, the time of application, and the distance the lamp is from the human body. Explicit instructions should accompany each lamp, and these instructions should be followed.

The infra-red lamp is for warming and easing an uncomfortable or painful part of the body; if properly applied it helps to overcome congestion so the blood can again flow freely. Of course, it is not curative, for the cure comes by purifying the body and rebuilding it with the right material. This is done by cleansing the body internally, and giving it plenty of water, the right foods, and good air—infra-red rays furnish nothing of this kind.

The sun lamp is used for its warm, tonic effect on the body. Great claims are made for it, and it is helpful, but it is no cure in rheumatism and arthritis. It does give the patient a lift, which is most desirable; the patient feels that something is done for him which raises his morale.

So if it is desired use either the infra-red or the sun lamp, but avoid overexposure, especially with the sun lamp. If burns occur, they may be difficult to heal. Even hot water bottles (rubber bags filled with hot water) put in the foot of the bed, and not sufficiently wrapped, have caused serious burns.

So beware and take care in handling all rays.

MEDICATION

The more we have seen of medication for rheumatism and arthritis the less we have liked it. Whether to take drugs for the relief of discomfort and pain involved is something to be decided by each patient. We are convinced that the drugging delays the recovery, for the body has to rid itself not only of its own accumulated toxins but of the poisonous drugs as well. And they are poisonous.

The most common of all drugs in arthritis, for decades, has been some compound known as a salicylate (a complex carbon-hydrogen-oxygen product.) Many doctors have told their patients, "It is harmless." But nay, nay, it is a poison. Give it in full dosage and it produces salicylism, a toxic condition in which the chief symptoms are ringing in the ears (tinnitus), nausea and vomiting, and the intellect is blunted (hebetude). Aspirin is the salicylate best known to lay persons, and it is not harmless. It is a sedative all right; it eases pain and dulls the mind and depresses the heart, and occasionally it kills someone, but who hears about that?

May we adduce some expert testimony, that of our Professor of Medicine, who believed so implicitly in the Materia Medica he long and faithfully taught: "We do not know what to do for arthritis; there is no known cure. But we use the salicylates, not that they do any good, but we have to give something or the patient will think he is being neglected, and small doses of the salicylates do no special harm."

But there is the cure of correct hygienic living, a cure that brings splendid results to those who do not wait until their joints are wrecked before adopting it.

And large doses of the salicylates poison the human body, occasionally to the point of death.

Nature cures.

12 Massage

This subject belongs in the chapter on treatments, but there is an important point we feel we must emphasize, and this we can best do by giving Massage a short chapter of its own.

The big question for an arthritic, or even a rheumatic is, should the painful parts be massaged. Some say yes, and others say no. As we have had successful experience in arthritis for over forty years, we feel our testimony is worth more than that given by those who have failed.

Ordinarily, massage is fine; it tones up the tissues; it helps to strengthen the muscles, it aids in normalizing the circulation, and is a blessing to many. But in certain conditions and locations massage can be torture that makes the illness worse.

Here are some facts from life: A gentleman over fifty years of age had such bad arthritis in the feet and ankles, also a little in the knees, that his walking was difficult—with each step he advanced about eight inches. Truth to tell, his hips were not

normal either. His physician believed in massage
in acute arthritis, and so he directed the masseur
to give the feet and ankles a good workout twice a
week; but this had to be reduced to once a week
because the patient became so painful he could
hardly take his mincing steps. Even with one massage a week he felt that he was losing ground,
walking more poorly as time went on.

So he quit that kind of treatment and placed himself in our care. We taught him how to eat and
drink and give himself hygienic care; we instructed
him to live as quietly as possible for a few weeks
and had him soak his feet and ankles in hot water
for twenty or more minutes, three times a week.
We also told him about soaking his knees and hips,
for his arms and shoulders were powerful enough
for him to enter and leave the bathtub. He gained
much ease during the first month; in the second
month he quit his mincing walk, regaining much
of his stride; in the next two months all soreness
left his feet and ankles. He was a good patient and
made a fine recovery. We have just had a letter
from him telling us that he has been in fine condition during the past year.

A WARNING ON JOINT MASSAGE

The big point we wish to make is this: Do not massage the afflicted joints, for it only irritates them
further.

But you may massage the fleshy part of the affected limb or limbs between the joints, not over the affected joints. Suppose the knee is badly arthritic; then massage the calf and the thigh, but not the knee. This is based on over forty years of observations; without exception, the affected joints have been made worse, when the joints themselves were massaged. There have been no bad results when the fleshy parts of the limbs have been massaged; in our judgment that has been helpful. The same is true of the arms and their joints.

We repeat, do not massage arthritic joints, but it is well to massage the fleshy part of the limbs between the joints.

What has been said of massage is also true of using any form of vibration—avoid doing it over the affected joints; also do not vibrate right over the spinal column, but you may vibrate on each side of the spine. This holds both in health and in disease, for the spine.

Again, treatments may be helpful, but they are not basic. The fundamental necessity in clearing up arthritis and rheumatism is right drinking, right eating, right inner cleansing of the body, and right constructive thinking.

13 A Day of Health Building

This chapter heading would have sounded odd years ago when we first became interested in health through natural living; nearly all then believed that it was necessary to take medicine to regain health. This belief began thousands of years ago, and still prevails among the majority. But now a large minority knows that we build disease by living wrong, as we build health by living right. And right living means to harmonize our lives with the great laws of Nature, which rule life. These laws are physical, mental (psychological), and spiritual.

For years our patients have tried to narrow them down to the rules for right eating—"it is all in the eating" we have repeatedly heard. But that is not true; there is much more to life and living than food and eating. We have to take all aspects of life into consideration; please remember that, always.

There are two fundamental points in rheumatic

and arthritic conditions that are of outstanding importance.

The first is to drink enough water to wash the impurities out of the body; these impurities are poisonous wastes that keep the body ill—or cause illness to appear. From the physical standpoint, the conquest of rheumatism and arthritis is the purification of the body. Water drinking is essential because water is the only fluid we have that washes the cells and carries the poisons out of the system by way of the skin, the lungs, the kidneys and the bowels. So every arthritic should drink enough water for this washing, purifying process of the inner body. A small woman needs five glasses of water daily (eight ounces to each glass of water), and a large man should drink about eight glasses of water daily. A rough rule is, drink a glass of water every day for every twenty pounds of body weight.

The second outstanding point is to lift up the mind—the thoughts and the emotions—and keep it on the constructive side. Certainly a person has to face reality; it is folly to be a Pollyanna, for that attitude is as false as the chronically depressive one. To lift up the mind means to recognize the good and favorable aspects of life; to appreciate them; and to be thankful for them; it means to face life in hope and confidence; it means to look ahead with the thought that improvement is to come.

Certainly it is unpleasant to be ill, but nothing is gained by going worrisome and depressive, by

becoming hopeless and whining—that attitude is a
mistake and a tragedy, for it makes conditions
worse, and in serious illness it may result in crippled joints and even in premature death.

THE MIND RULES THE BODY

It is difficult to explain the effect of the mind, which
includes the emotions, on the body. But the mind
rules the body. When the mind is calm, as it should
be most of the time, it helps the body to relax and
function normally. When depressive thoughts and
emotions rule the mind, the body becomes de-
pressed; it tightens up, and this helps to upset the
emotions even more. When a certain amount of
tightening takes place, we call it tension. The more
tension, the more the functions of the body are
upset. Tension is one cause of the evil we call
constipation. Depression and tension upset the
nervous system, and quickly play havoc with the
digestion, which, we repeat, results in bad blood
and disease.

And one direct result of depression and tension
is the manufacture of toxins within the body; this
has been scientifically established; just how it happens is not clear, but it is a well established fact. As
autointoxication, or the toxic state, is the basic
cause of arthritis, the evil results of depression and
tension are self-evident.

Please remember that the term nervous tension is misleading, for the tension is primarily of the mind, resulting when the mind is in turmoil; so it is necessary to keep the mind's house in order; it is mental tension, not nervous tension, that is back of mental upsets and depressions; it is mental tension that helps to poison us into arthritis.

Another fact to remember is that those who have arthritis do not usually recover in a steady progression; they have their ups and downs. So long as there is arthritic poison in the body, a temporary upset can occur. Also, although many arthritics lose their bad symptoms in one, or two, or three months, not all do so. Some who still have the ability to recover require a year or more for the symptoms to fade away. Of course, there are those who are so badly wrecked that recovery is impossible, although most of them can gain freedom from pain.

Impatience retards progress. "Doctor, I still have arthritis," said a woman at the end of three days of supervision, and numerous patients have said it at the end of two or three weeks. This is not only lack of patience, but lack of understanding. It is true that most of our arthritics, treated as here recommended, have gained comfort in three months or less, but that is not possible for all. We have been consulted by a few in such bad condition that they were prisoners of wheel chairs; most of them have been happy to get rid of their pains, and a part of their deformities in a year; they also gained some mobility. No one should permit disease to get such a terrible hold. But despite this, please remember that the great majority can rid themselves of arthritis if they have the will.

A HEALTH-BUILDING DAY

1   On first arising in the morning, wash and rinse the mouth well with water; if you wish to add a little salt, or sodium bicarbonate, or lemon juice, or tooth paste to do the cleansing, very good; brushing the teeth is a part of the cleansing process.

The reason for cleaning the mouth before eating and drinking in the morning is that bacteria abound in the mouth; they throw out their own wastes or toxins, and it is best not to swallow big doses of this material.

After the mouth is well cleansed, drink one or two glasses of water. This is helpful because water taken in this way is a gentle laxative.

If the plan is to have starch in the breakfast, it is a good idea to sip a glass of orange or grapefruit juice at the water drinking time on first arising. The reason is that those who have inferior digestion do better if both starch and fruit juice are not taken during the same meal. Then it is best to wait at least thirty minutes after the fruit juice sipping before taking a starchy meal. If the digestion is superb, starch and acid may be taken in the same meal.

2 If you are able to take exercises, the best time is after drinking the morning liquid, for that adds to the natural laxative tendency. Exercises and exercising will be discussed elsewhere in this volume. But one thing we wish to emphasize: Do no violent exercises in arthritis, and be gentle with the affected joint. This is one disease where injudicious exercises can do much harm. Here is an example:

A middle-aged woman was making a beautiful recovery from arthritis; she had attained the point where she had lost all aches, all pains, all soreness; her body was easy. She was strongly warned not to attempt any hard work or prolonged application to any task. But there was a big ironing to do the following Tuesday, and the laundress did not show up. So our patient ironed the whole day long, and "it felt so good to be able to work like that once more." The next day powerful pains returned, and it took many weeks to regain comfort.

This time she gave her joints a fair chance; her recovery was splendid, and she told us a short time ago that she was remained well and active during the intervening twelve years.

3 All the preparations have been made, and the patient is ready for

BREAKFAST

A glass of orange juice, either now
    or at water drinking time
Baked apple, core stuffed with soaked raisins
If still hungry, add some sweet plums
At end of meal slowly sip a glass of milk

And please remember to eat in peace and amity at every meal, for when the mind is calm and friendly the digestion is at its best. And another reminder: Please eat slowly at your breakfast, lunch and dinner 365 days a year—always—please, please, please.

4   Either after the exercise, or within thirty minutes after the breakfast, go to the bathroom and give the intestines a chance to function—do this whether there is any call or not, for this is one of the measures that helps to regain lost bowel function, that is, regularly soliciting a bowel function at a certain time each day; we have often seen this referred to as habit-time.

Not only is water drunk by itself or with fruit juice on first arising in the morning a gentle intestinal tonic, but food itself stimulates action in the intestines, so we can truly call food a mild laxative —that is why we tie up bowel functioning with water drinking and meals.

And a clean bowel is a basic necessity in overcoming rheumatism and arthritis.

5 You drank water on arising; maybe you drank water at the beginning or end of the breakfast; a very good time to drink more water is the middle of the forenoon; and still another excellent time is the middle of the afternoon. Be sure to get your quota of water every day—five glasses if you are a small person; six or seven if you are medium-sized; eight glasses if you are large. You will find more about this elsewhere in the book. This is just a summary of a living-for-health day. It requires plenty of water to wash the toxins out of the body, the poisons that are such a great factor in causing rheumatism and arthritis.

6 Either in the forenoon or afternoon, go out for fresh air and sunshine whenever the weather permits. Details will be found elsewhere in this book. But please remember that fresh air, day and night, is most helpful, for it furnishes the needed oxygen to the blood, without having to inhale harmful fumes and grime so common in our cities. Of all physical needs, fresh air is the most essential, for we are unable to live more than about four minutes without the precious oxygen.

And sunlight! It is the source and origin of all the high life on earth; plants and animals could not exist without it; human life could not exist without it. Take away the sun, and our cunning little earth would turn dark and so cold that every sign of higher life would soon vanish. So let the sun shine upon your body and thus manufacture in the most natural way a good supply of vitamin D. If you are not used to sunshine on your body surfaces, expose them to the sunlight not more than five minutes the first day, that is, each surface; and then slowly increase until the various body surfaces receive about fifteen minutes of sunlight—this would require about an hour daily.

But let all with fair skin remember that overexposure to sunshine is bad; it may induce weakness, blood deterioration and even death. We well remember a healthy young woman, fair of coloration, who thought she could not get enough of Texas sunshine; she remained in the midday sunshine even on the hottest days, every fair day. Her excessive sun worship ended her life while she was much too young to die.

7 And now it is time for the midday meal, but before we plan that, let us remember a very important point for all meals. Salt is essential to health, but there is a tendency among many to overseason, not only with salt but with spices. Salt helps to retain fluids within the body, but when the salt intake is excessive, the fluid retention tends to be excessive too. This prevents the rapid elimination of poisonous waste. So use salt sparingly. This is important in arthritis, and all other toxin-induced diseases, but of course it is even more important in arteriosclerosis.

LUNCH

Vegetable soup, no crackers, no meat stock
Head lettuce, tomato slices, avocado strips
Large dish of Swiss chard, or green string beans
Whole wheat-raisin toast, butter
Fresh ripe peaches with cream

Again, vegetables are the most important of all foods in overcoming arthritis, which is our reason for using them so freely in lunches and dinners.

8 Overeating is to be avoided. Some human beings eat repeatedly between meals, and they taste foods while preparing them for the table. This must be avoided. Do not permit overweight—see discussion on this subject in another chapter.

The only food permitted between meals is mild fresh fruit, such as melons, blueberries, pears, peaches, apricots, mild apples, and other fruits that are mild but full of juice. To make it emphatic, no breads, no meats, no cakes or cookies, no milk, no cheese—nothing between meals except fresh mild fruit, and the only time should be in midafternoon. No food before retiring at night.

DINNER

French endive with ripe olives
Green peas and broccoli

Baked or jacket-cooked yams
Roast leg of lamb
Baked bananas

Unsweetened apple sauce goes with leg of lamb, if desired. It may be flavored with mint. If a salad of mixed vegetables is preferred to endive and olives, make the change. If you would rather have other vegetables than peas and broccoli, very well —spinach and carrots, for instance. Always try to have one vegetable that is green in color in the dinner. Yes, the color green means added vitality in the food.

9 If the intestines have not functioned during the day, be sure they do so during the evening, and a good time is within thirty or forty minutes after dinner, while the food stimulation is still at work on stomach and intestines.

10 If the patient is able to get in and out of the bathtub, the bath may be taken at any time in the day, but not soon after meals—it is all right to bathe before meals, or about three hours after meals. In arthritis avoid cold water as much as possible. Warm water is more soothing, and a greater help in equalizing the circulation; cold water often brings pain in rheumatism and arthritis, while warm water often relieves the pain.

It is the warm water that helps in arthritis, not necessarily anything added to the water; but there is no harm in dissolving a glass or a little more of Epsom salts in a tub of bath water.

If the hips, or the knees and ankles are painful, it is a good idea to draw eight or ten inches of water as hot as the body can comfortably bear in the bathtub, and sit in the tub for about 15 minutes while the legs soak.

If unable to use the tub, the patient should take a shower bath or have the body surfaces sponged enough to remain clean.

Some arthritics have considerable itching; they should use the purest of soap in great moderation and wash the soap away with plenty of clear rinsing water. Rubbing a little oil into the skin after the bath relieves dryness and tends to help the itching. As acidity is generally excessive in arthritis, dry and itching skin is rather common.

After the bath it is always well to give the skin some dry friction with a firm bath towel or a rubbing mitt that is not coarse enough to hurt the skin; the palms are also good for body rubs. The rubbing is tonic to the surface, circulation included.

Many of our patients have carried on their work while recovering from rheumatism and arthritis. They have found the time to take care of themselves, but the work has interfered with airing in the sun and walks—if able to walk—in daylight hours. They may of course use the sun lamp, finding out how long they should expose themselves to its rays so as to avoid burning.

Various treatments will be discussed in another chapter, but please remember that correct living, physically and mentally, is the best treatment of all, the only treatment on which we can rely.

14 Your Own Attitude Toward Arthritis

So you have arthritis. The way you use your mind, your attitude, will almost surely determine whether you are to recover or sink deeper and deeper into the disease.

If you believe the old fallacy that arthritis is incurable and give up, you will almost certainly become a prisoner of the disease. But if you tell yourself that you are going to do your best to overcome it, get the correct knowledge, and live that knowledge, you will almost surely recover. A few let the disease become so severe, with completely wrecked joints, that mobility of those joints refuses to return. But even they can generally regain freedom from pain and ease of body.

Suppose you have rheumatoid arthritis in acute form (as described in another chapter), are you to reason that because you have a remission, you are well? That would be a mistake, for after a while

149

a more severe attack usually occurs, and after a number of these acute attacks, chronic rheumatoid arthritis establishes itself. We have elsewhere told you the story of the Canadian woman who deceived herself and evaded the issue until she became a cripple.

STORIES WITH HAPPY ENDINGS

Let us tell you the story of a woman who had rather severe rheumatoid arthritis. She went to a specialist in her city, a man who unfortunately thought that arthritis was incurable. He told his patient that "There is no cure for arthritis. Your joints are already a little deformed (arthritis deformans). This will continue and you will become stiffer with the passing years. The best you can do is to get yourself a wheel chair and assume a comfortable position, with arms and legs flexed, or go to bed and take the easiest position you can find. It is better to stiffen up that way than to have the limbs straight."

She went to bed, face to the wall. This is a position of defeat and despair which we have encountered in a few patients who had given up all attempts to recover, not only in arthritis but in other ills. One man gambled in Wall Street when almost no margin was required, lost all of his money, and went to bed, face to the wall. His recovery, after he heard a few truths, was so sudden that it was comical.

The woman who lost all hope had a wealthy brother who refused to accept the incurable verdict. He told her to change doctors, and we had the pleasure of instilling hope in her mind, of getting her to arise from bed, and in the course of a few months of returning to complete usefulness, again able to take physical care of her aged mother. We knew the whole family, so we can testify that she continued in good health for many years. Her hands were not as pretty as a woman would like, but the swelling, and much of the deformity, vanished.

It is obvious that this patient could not have recovered as long as she despaired, for in that state of mind she could not have followed the simple but fundamental directions about eating and drinking right, and the needed hygienic care.

One woman we found in a wheel chair with legs and feet rigidly fixed; her arms were crossed on her chest, the fingers fixed and extended. The verdict had been that she was ankylosed and would never be able to use them again. She had slight mobility in shoulders and neck, so with considerable effort she could touch her hands to her chin, but not to her face. After carefully sizing her up we told her: "Some of your joints are limed up (ankylosed) and their movement is lost. But more of the joints are held rigid by pain; you can regain the motion in these joints, and experience says you can lose the pain."

She had the right spirit and replied: "I shall do everything I can to regain as much lost ground as possible." And she did. She regained the ability of moving her feet freely, and after a few months she could bring her hands to her face, very important for a woman who had a young grandson who did not understand that he should keep the screen door closed. It had been trying for the grandmother to have the flies settle on her face without the ability to drive them away. Furthermore, she was able to do a rather good job of putting up her own hair. Although she was partly disabled she never complained—she was a wonderful woman. She lived in comfort until pneumonia ended her life at the age of seventy-two years, in comfort and in good cheer.

A TALE OF FAILURE

But it is not always a tale of victory. A gentleman who was imprisoned in his home with arthritis said he wanted to get rid of as much arthritis as possible. He was in bad condition, somewhat like that of the cheerful woman whose tale we have just told. He could have made the same kind of partial recovery that she did. But he was completely negative, full of worry, fear and depression—so far as

arthritis was concerned, his attitude was completely destructive.

We explained to him repeatedly that he had to
lift up his mind, that he had to develop the expect-
ancy of betterment, that he had to hope for improvement, that he had to hope that if he treated
himself right, the arthritis would lessen. We failed
to make any impression on him, and as soon as we
were convinced that he would not give up his depression and despair, we discharged ourselves. He
had means, and he even paid other arthritics to
come to his home to discuss with him the hopelessness and the incurability of arthritis. It was a mania
with him. One of his relatives was a patient, and
years later he informed us that he continued to
steep himself in the hopelessness of arthritis. So
this was an abject failure.

RAPID RECOVERY AT 70 PLUS

Just one more brief illustration of attitude towards
arthritis. A woman over seventy years of age began
with these remarks, "I suppose my time of free activity is finished; it is so painful to walk and work
or play, and my movements are limited; as I am
over seventy years of age, I have been told repeatedly that I have had my day. But I know two of
your recovered patients, so I am here to make my
final effort." We explained to her that recovery is

not dependent on the age of the individual, but on the amount of vitality he is able to summon in his endeavors to recover. Also, we impressed on her that she had to be patient, for after seventy the recovery is slower than in younger years.

She was an excellent patient. As soon as she lost a part of her pain her mental attitude became as hopeful and positive as any doctor could desire. She had good vitality, so she astonished us by losing her aches, pains, soreness and stiffness in about half of the time our experience had led us to expect—in less than three months. After that she continued to live right so as to eliminate all the toxicity of her body, thus preventing the return of the disability and pain of arthritis. Yes, she has remained well.

Our experience with thousands of arthritics is this: Those who cooperate physically by living hygienically, and mentally by acquiring a confident, hopeful, courageous outlook, as regards arthritis and life in general are elevated in body and mind to the point where they are in favorable condition for healing. They make good recoveries, unless they have permitted the disease to go to such extremes that Nature refuses to forgive.

Those who let fear, worry, apprehension and anxiety—Horace Fletcher called these the cowardly emotions—rule them, usually give up the effort to recover. Instead of graduating into good health, they usually quituate into worry, depression and continued disease.

ALL UP TO YOU

So how are you to direct your thoughts and emotions—into negative, depressive ways that lead to permanent disease? Or into hopeful, confident, courageous and constructive channels that bring recovery with the possibility of success and satisfaction in living?

It is up to you.

We have told tales from life of those who recovered and of those who failed. Those who recovered lived physically and mentally as we recommend in this book. And that brings a repetition of the fact that merely reading this book does no good; one has to live these teachings to receive the benefits. The other day we received a letter from a patient who some years ago recovered from the disease for which he consulted us. He ended with, "I cannot understand why I am so badly crippled with rheumatism that I had to give up my law practice, for I have continued to do some of the things you taught me about right living." Of course, the solution was easy—he did too many things wrong.

To be healthy we have to live healthfully, not merely play at it.

15 Vegetables in Arthritis

In the final chapter on Food and Cooking we list many foods including numerous vegetables, but by no means all that are available in the market.

In arthritis the vegetables are the most important of all of the foods, for they help to alkalize the body; they bring an abundance of organic mineral salts into the system; they contain vitamins, and they have a helpful effect on the intestines, strongly tending towards bowel regularity and internal cleanliness.

But here is the rub: Many patients object, "I get so tired of vegetables, it is so monotonous to have them every day." One man who wanted beefsteak, French-fried potatoes and apple pie for dinner every day, and often had the same meal for lunch, until he suffered not only with arthritis but with hypertension as well, made this complaint.

We answered as follows: "You have been eating

steak daily, if you could obtain it; that wasn't monotonous. You have eaten fried potatoes and apple pie several hundred times a year, and that wasn't monotonous. Finally this unbalanced, unwholesome food plan, aided by mental tension, made you ill. Much as you loved those foods they were not your friends. They helped to put you where you are, in a condition where you are unable to carry on your business. On the other hand, the vegetables are friendly to you; they will help to restore you to good enough health so you can return to your activities, and there are dozens of them, so there is no reason why you should tire of them. You have to make up your mind what you want, to destroy yourself with foods and drinks and mental tensions that are inimical to your health, or take the foods, drinks and mental attitude that aid in restoring you to better health and usefulness."

Whether or not we like a food is largely the result of habit. Happy are they who cultivate the habit of eating wholesome foods.

USE IMAGINATION IN COOKING

To those who prepare food for the sick, or prescribe food plans, let us say: Use your imagination in cooking. Avoid the bad habit of selecting corn, carrots and peas, and string beans for the meals day after day. Use variety in planning, not only in cooked vegetables but in salads, and prepare some of them in different ways.

Take the onion as an illustration: Usually it is stewed, which is all right; but it may be cooked half onion sliced and half tomato; or one-third each of onion, tomato and sliced okra; or it may be peeled, sliced and broiled; or it may be peeled, cut crosswise into halves and baked; or it may form a part of vegetable soup; or it may be sliced and served with lettuce and lemon—raw onion; or it may be cut fine and mixed with the salad or a little minced onion may be put in the salad dressing; the fleshy stem of the scallions may be cut four or five inches long and cooked like asparagus—it is delicate and delicious. And the onion may be dressed with butter or genuine cream (not with the so-called cream sauce) or with oil, and salt in moderation. This is just a beginning for onion goes well with cut-up or chopped meats, and in meat loaves. Use your imagination.

Take the prosaic beet: Its tender leaves make a delicious dish of cooking greens—cooked like spinach; the tender beet stalks, diced, make a good vegetable; it is even better if you mix the stalks with greens; the beet roots are good when cooked tender; but the best dish of all is when you cook and dice the beet root, and add to it the diced stalks and the tender beet greens and mix. It's a dish fit for the king and the queen too, and very good for rheumatics and arthritics.

When it comes to selecting vegetables for the dinner or lunch, avoid the practice of relying on only a few kinds. We recommend two cooked vegetables in every dinner, as you will see by looking at the numerous menus we have given you in this book. Let us plan the cooked dinner vegetables for a week, maybe using one favorite vegetable, and one that is not so well known to the lady of the house, or at least that is green in color, and please remember that the cooked vegetables are the most valuable, the cooking greens.

1 Baked carrot strips and Swiss chard.
2 Green young lima beans and scallions cooked like asparagus.
3 String beans and beet greens with diced beet stalks.
4 Green peas and broccoli cooked with tender leaves.
5 Stewed baby onions and green asparagus tips.
6 Corn on the cob and okra stewed with tomatoes.
7 Stewed celery and cone artichoke.

Monotonous? Certainly not. Interesting and delicious? Surely. Use your imagination and you will have the best of foods.

VEGETABLE SALAD

It is the same way with salads. Use your imagination and vary them; also vary the dressing. Yes, use your imagination; sometimes use some fruit for the sake of change. For instance, most persons use oil and vinegar on every salad; we advise the omission of the vinegar for the living citrus acid of lemon or lime juice. But sometimes omit these, and use orange sections or grapefruit sections, membranes removed, to furnish the salad acidity. Also, we use the avocado, full of oil, as the oily dressing of the salad—no, we use no oil when we have avocado in the salad. Also, the tomato contains its own acid, so when we have plenty of tomato in the salad, we use no other acid. Let us illustrate:

Make a foundation of tender lettuce leaves, place thereon tomato slices and over them avocado strips; it looks fine and tastes better. No dressing needed.

Many years ago we knew well and worked with a very fine physician, Dr. J. H. Tilden, of Denver, Colorado. He made up a salad of lettuce, tomatoes and cucumbers, flavored with onions, and called it the Tilden salad. When he planned dinners for his patients he would always include the "Tilden Salad." It is good but not good enough to be exclusive. For the sake of interest let there be imagination and variety in salads. Here are some, always simple, for the more different ingredients in the salad, the more difficult it is to digest.

1 Lettuce, sliced tomatoes, chopped cabbage and pimiento strips.

2 French endive, sliced cucumbers, grated carrot mounds and ripe olives.

3 Green lettuce, grated turnips, avocado strips and orange sections.

4 The Tilden salad—lettuce, tomatoes and cucumbers with enough onion for flavoring.

5 Chopped young cabbage on lettuce with avocado strips.

6 Romaine, heart of celery and sliced tomatoes.

7 Celery cabbage, sliced cucumbers, avocado and strips of pimiento. (Cut celery cabbage across the grain.)

8 Chicory, tomatoes, diced apple and avocado.

9 Lettuce, celery, grapefruit sections, with pimiento strips and watercress.

10 Endive, tomato, avocado strips and watercress.

Some like very simple salads, and all they need is one raw vegetable, such as a wedge of head lettuce, with or without avocado; a plate of sliced tomato and nothing else; or a plate of cucumbers, in strips or slices; or tender young celery, with or without ripe olives. Strips of green peppers are fine with salads.

Green peppers, cut in strips or diced, are also good cooked with other vegetables, such as onions, or tomatoes, or string beans.

And mushrooms add a pleasant flavor to vegetables; they should be cut up and added towards the end of the cooking, so they will not be cooked overlong. But if we continue this, the chapter will be overlong. Please remember, by varying the vegetables from day to day, and using a little wit and imagination, the vegetables become one of the most pleasant and attractive parts of the meal. In the last dinner we gave, one of the guests remarked, the salad is what I shall remember, and it was so simple: On a bed of French endive, we place some fat slices of beefsteak tomatoes, over that strips of avocados, and on top a few slim cheddar cheese sticks—but the tomatoes were of a quality not expected in winter. The asparagus and tiny white onions also came in for favorable comment—in our home the vegetables star.

FRUIT AND VEGETABLE DIET

We have repeatedly said the fruits, vegetables and water are the compounds that alkalize and cleanse the body, hence help to build health. Then why not adopt a fruit and vegetable diet? Yes, why not? For those who are well fleshed, it is a wonderful plan, for at least a week or two. For those who are slender, and either arthritic or rheumatic, it would be good to live one or two days a week on nothing but fruits, vegetables and water. Of course, no one is able to live on such a plan indefinitely, for the fruits and vegetables would not furnish enough protein.

For those who are well fleshed a good plan for overcoming arthritis is to live three days each week on nothing but fruits, vegetables and water; the rest of the time live as outlined elsewhere in this book, where you will find plenty of menus.

In selecting the vegetables, be sure to have one that is green in color, one that is leafy, in every meal, for the green leaves are richer in organic mineral salts, vitamins and chlorophyll than any other parts of the vegetables—young green cabbage, broccoli, Swiss chard, beet tops, turnip tops, collards—the broccoli is to be cooked with the tender young leaves, which are delicious—not with the big, coarse leaves. Such greens, and other favorite ones, are the best medicine we have for arthritis.

As for the fruits: Select the ones that are full of juice as you bite into them, but if painful avoid the fruits that are very tart, except that once a day you take a portion of oranges or grapefruit—enough to make a glass of juice. Take melons plentifully, berries in season, pears, apples, peaches, apricots—all juicy fruits, and there are others.

Let us demonstrate:

BREAKFAST

Either oranges or grapefruit
What melons you desire
Pears

LUNCH

A salad of lettuce and tomato
Beet tops with diced beet stems
Carrots with minced green pepper
Cherries

DINNER

Celery-apple-avocado salad
Young spinach cooked with minced onion
Young green lima beans
Either ripe banana or fresh ripe figs

And that is all; be very sparing with all dressings, which have been explained elsewhere; be
especially sparing with fats and oils, and dressings
made of oil, for these are heavy foods, and if much
of them is consumed, it interferes with the cleansing action of the water, vegetables and fruit. However, do not overeat, for that upsets the digestion,
and thus makes inferior blood which is no help to
rheumatics. Plenty of water, please.

OVEREATING

Overeating is one of the greatest of evils, especially
in this land of plenty. What we need and eat sus-

tains us and helps us to be healthy; what we eat beyond that builds disease.

To avoid overeating:

1 Be calm, pleasant and kind at meal times—never correct the children or anyone else during the meals; never engage in heated arguments at this time.

2 Always eat very slowly and masticate well at every meal—always.

3 Avoid drinking during the meal—no liquids with the solid foods. But you may drink at the beginning of the meal and at the end of the meal.

4 For emphasis, never hurry, never rush at meal times. You have all the time there is, all the time anyone has—twenty-four hours each day.

5 The minute you feel you have had enough, stop eating. Never, never, never eat until feeling full and stuffy and even uncomfortable.

Yes, always be a moderate eater for that is one of the paths of health.

16 Foods That Build Health

The general attitude towards foods has been that so long as they are filling, give heat and energy, while repairing the waste of the living process, nothing more matters. But foods have another great function, and that is to build health.

For the purposes of producing heat and energy, and performing the essential repairs, we might live on white sugar and its products, white flour and its products, with the addition of a little fat, and some fried meat to give the body its essential nitrogen. But such a food plan would soon produce disease. Why? Because white sugar is a dead carbon food devoid of vitamins and the needed mineral salts; white flour is a partly devitalized food; fried meats are largely spoiled in the cooking. These foods lack the vital elements, or compounds, which we speak of as organic mineral salts and the vitamins, which we may call body activators or conditioners. Those who have a true desire to recover from arthritis should avoid white sugar, white flour and its products and all fried foods.

Honey and maple sugar and maple syrup, also brown sugar, are good sweeteners; so are raisins, figs and dates; sweet prunes are high in sugar; about one-fifth of the ripe banana is sugar. Instead of eating white bread and other white flour products, take whole wheat bread or other whole flour or whole grain products, for these contain the vitamins and mineral salts so largely lost in producing the white flour.

MINERAL SALTS DEFINED

What are the mineral salts of which we speak? They are the compounds of minerals and metals needed by the body to perform their function. Many realize that calcium or lime is essential to health, for the dairy companies have kept the public well informed on this point and the fact that milk is rich in lime. Where did the cow get all of that lime? From the grass on which she fed. Where may we obtain it if we are unable to eat milk—yes, milk is a food so we may correctly say we eat it. We may also obtain lime by eating our form of grass—raw vegetable salads and the leafy vegetables. The vegetable leaves are rich in not only lime, but in iron and other metals and minerals, also in vitamins, also in chlorophyll, the green wonder chemical of Nature, which makes food growing possible. Except that its basis is not iron, chlorophyll is almost the same as the hemoglobin, so essential to the blood and our very ability to live.

By the way, milk is impoverished in iron, which is as necessary to our lives as lime. Milk is a good food, but not an essential one for adults. This is a good thing, for a few millions of our population are so badly catarrhal that they should not take milk— milk makes the catarrh (manifesting in many acute and chronic colds) worse.

We also need the salts of potash and sodium; we need compounds of sulphur and phosphorus; we need ever so many of these salts, including a trace of copper and boron. But it is not our aim to write a chemical treatise. The basic truth one should remember is to take foods that contain their original supply of these mineral salts. This can be done by avoiding highly refined foods, the worst of all being white sugar and its products; white flour and its products are not quite as bad, but they are bad enough so they should be omitted from the food plan. Frying is bad because it makes the foods hard to digest, and spoils the parts turned into a crisp crust.

Another way of spoiling foods rich in vital elements is to cook vegetables in much water, and pour the cooking liquor down the drain, thus losing the health values; also, peeling potatoes and then cooking them, thus losing the best part of this good food. Cook the vegetables in very little water, and consume your share of the cooking liquor; bake your potatoes, or boil or steam or pressure cook them in the peel (or jacket).

BE MODERATE IN VITAMIN DOSAGES

There is a great tendency for human beings to go to extremes. One woman on learning that organic mineral salts and vitamins are essential to health decided to fortify herself so well with these compounds that she would surely remain well. So she went to a specialty food shop and purchased thirty-two different kinds of mineral compounds and vitamins and specially enriched foods, and made up a plan to consume some of each compound every day —with the result that she developed a bad case of indigestion, and enough gas pressure in the region of the heart to believe she had heart disease. When she first consulted us, she brought a bag containing her specialty products, displaying all thirty-two of them on our desk.

The end of the story is that she had no heart disease, only excessive gas pressure in that region, largely induced by trying to eat too many remedial foods at each meal—she had no indigestion until she started to eat herself into assured health with specialty products. Of course, we have no objec-

tion to vitamins and mineral salts and good specialty products within reason, but it is always a
mistake to go to extremes in taking vitamins and
mineral salts. It is always a mistake to take large
quantities of vitamins, or massive doses of them
without the advice of a doctor who knows what he
is talking about. Excessive dosing with some vitamins can produce disease—seeing such patients
reminds us how good was the ancient Greek saying
of "nothing too much." We say, moderation in all
things, and we might add that enough is plenty.
Excess in any physical line leads to disease.

IDEAL DIET SUPPLIES ALL VITAMINS

What is the practical truth about vitamins and mineral salts for the sake of health? It is that these
compounds are contained in the good foods on the
market, foods grown on good soil and not spoiled
in the cooking.

Those who eat freely of raw salads, cooked vegetables, raw fruits and cooked fruits, some milk, butter or good substitute, potatoes cooked in the jacket, whole wheat or other whole grain bread, and
meat, with eggs twice a week, get every mineral
salt needed by the body and every essential vitamin. If they further take the precaution of eating
salt-water fish—fish from the ocean—once or twice

a week, they make asurance doubly sure. The reason is that for ages the sea has been robbing the land of its soluble mineral contents, so the sea contains plants and animals well stocked with these precious health compounds; much fish that is not eaten is used for fertilizer, and good fertilizer it is. For instance, the iodine has been washed out of much of the soil in mountains and other well drained areas; as a result, those who live there are apt to have goitre unless they take salt or foods containing iodine—this is reason for iodized table salt. The sea and its creatures are rich in iodine.

Please remember the basic truth that those who daily eat good unspoiled foods get all the health elements they need—vitamins and organic mineral salts. But let us illustrate this point with menus for a day:

BREAKFAST

Glass of orange juice (30 minutes before rest of meal)
Sweet pears, best taken raw
Whole wheat raisin toast, butter
Glass of milk, if desired

The orange juice is rich in vitamin C, giving all that is needed for the day, but there is vitamin C in other fruits too, and in some vegetables—fresh cabbage contains as much as the orange juice. The oranges contain other vitamins and many mineral salts. So do the pears.

The whole wheat is rich in various vitamin B compounds, also in vitamin E. Butter contains vitamin A and probably carotene, a precursor of vitamin A.

And the milk is a good source of vitamins A and D.

NATURAL VITAMIN SOURCES

This would be a good place to give you a summary of the most prominent origins of the various vitamins:

Vitamin A is freely present in fishliver oils, eggs, butter, liver and cream, and of course in milk. Carotene, which the body has the power to turn into vitamin A, is abundant in carrots, other yellow and orange colored vegetables, and in the green leaves of vegetables—the leafy greens.

Vitamin B-1 (thiamine hydrochloride) is present in many vegetables, eggs, legumes, whole grains, and grain germs, liver, other meats and yeast.

Vitamin B-2 (riboflavin) is present in whole wheat, wheat germ, liver, milk, yeast, eggs, leafy vegetables, meat, legumes—peas, beans and lentils.

Niacin or nicotinic acid, also in the B group, is freely present in liver, meat and animal organs, whole grains including whole wheat and wheat germ and the leafy vegetables.

B-6 (pyridoxine hydrochloride) is found in whole wheat, whole rice, wheat germ, rice germ, sugar cane, liver and yeast.

Folic acid, also in the B group, is found in yeast, liver, other animal organs. Smaller amounts are present in many leafy vegetables, whole grains including the germ, also in meats and fish.

Please remember that the B vitamins are present in fish, one of the best sources of both vitamins and organic mineral salts—fish from the ocean.

Truth to tell, you eat the foods where these vitamins are found and you get B-12, helpful in blood conditioning.

Vitamin C (ascorbic acid) is abundant in citrus fruit—oranges, lemons, grapefruit and limes; also in tomatoes, fresh strawberries; new cabbage freshly cut, green peppers and other fruits and vegetables, especially the leafy ones.

Vitamin D presents itself in milk, cream and butter; also in eggs, liver and fish oils made of fish liver. This vitamin is also created when the sun shines on the skin, turning ergesterol in the body into this vitamin.

Vitamin E is present in most foods; it is almost impossible to run short of it if the eating is at least fairly good. It abounds in meat, eggs, green leafy vegetables, whole wheat and wheat germ. Eat right and there is no need of taking wheat germ oil.

Vitamin K, a blood conditioner, is found in liver, soybeans, cabbage, tomatoes, spinach, kale and other vegetables.

GENERAL ADVICE ON DIET

This is only a summary, but surely it has the moral that we should eat plenty of green leafy vegetables, not only cooked but raw; that we should eat fruit in abundance—there are more vitamins in fruits than indicated in the summary; that we should avoid refined flour, but take whole grain foods; that we should have fish regularly; that we should take several eggs each week, and have broiled or baked (not fried) liver once a week, and take meat once a day if we do not have fish or eggs that day. Please remember that fish is a surer source of both vitamins and organic mineral salts than meat. The text books are apt to dwell much on wheat germ oil and fishliver oil; what we should stress is the eating of fish at least once or twice per week, and take whole wheat bread, which includes the wheat germ, and avoid all products made of white flour.

LUNCH

Sliced tomatoes with avocado strips
Swiss chard cooked with cut chives
Baked potatoes with butter
Sliced bananas with cream

There you have more vitamin C in the tomatoes, with plenty of fat in the avocado; the Swiss chard is one of the greens, rich in vitamins as shown in the summary we have just given; the bananas contain many vitamin B compounds and the cream furnishes vitamins A and D, while Vitamin E is present in most foods.

ORGANIC MINERAL SALTS

Let us now consider the organic mineral salts, so called because they have been organized by the vegetable kingdom so that those in the animal kingdom, man included, may use them. Not long ago we found the statement in a great reference book that we need pay no attention to the mineral salts, except those of iron and calcium (lime), for if they are present, the other essential ones are there too. There is some truth in this statement, but it is not the truth. For instance, iron and lime in the soil and consequently in the food may be sufficient after the iodine has been leached out of the soil; so there is not enough iodine left for human health in the food grown on that soil.

The remedy is simple: Eat correctly prepared ocean fish twice a week and the body will obtain enough of not only iodine, but of the trace minerals, such as copper and boron, to maintain physical health. No one is certain how many elements are needed by the human body, but probably twenty or more of them are necessary, and all of these are in the ocean, from which the fish obtains them—from that nourishing broth that is the sea.

It would be interesting to observe what are the foods that furnish a goodly amount of iron:

The chief iron foods are chard, beet greens, spinach, turnip greens, kale, lettuce leaves—so far all of them leafy greens. Also dried peas and beans, liver and oysters; also whole wheat bread and meat, eggs, baked potatoes, raisins and oatmeal—the whole grain foods, not the refined white flour and foods made therefrom.

The chief lime foods are beet greens, broccoli, cauliflower, chard, mustard greens, kale, and spinach—so far all of them are leafy greens; milk and cottage cheese; also dried beans and dried figs—this is by no means a complete list. But we wish to repeat that if too catarrhal to eat milk and cheese, we may obtain our supply of calcium from the same source as the cow—the leafy greens.

And please note that white sugar has not once been referred to as the source of vitamins or organic mineral salts—the white sugar is too dead to contain the health food values, which is the greatest reason for avoiding this common article of food, which has nothing to offer to the human body except heat and energy, at the expense of health. It makes rheumatism and arthritis worse.

Although refined white flour has a little of the vital health elements in it, it is so small that we do not refer to it as a source of health supply. Rheumatics and arthritics should taboo the foods made of or with white flour.

For both vitamins and mineral salts, let us illustrate with a

DINNER

Salad of lettuce, tomatoes and ripe olives
Spinach cooked with minced green peppers
Green colored young lima beans
Steamed scrod (baby cod) with butter sauce
Dessert: Baked apple with cream

There you have everything: In the lettuce and spinach you have A and B and C—more C in the

tomatoes; in the scrod you have A and B and D—
more A and D in the cream—surely, the lima beans
and the baked apples add to the procession of the
first part of the alphabet, and if you have a keen
eye, you will find K emerging from the green peppers and elsewhere.

And this dinner is loaded with mineral salts, not
only iron and lime, but sodium, potash, sulphur,
phosphorus and all the rest needed by the body.
The greatest carriers of the organic mineral salts
are the lettuce, spinach and scrod—in this dinner.
But every food is vital; every food here is not only
nourishing but health-building. It is what is needed
in arthritic disease to vanquish this destroyer of
physical beauty and usefulness.

We are surely justified in repeating:

"Those who eat freely of raw salads, cooked
vegetables, raw fruits and cooked fruits, some milk,
butter or a good substitute, potatoes cooked in the
jacket, whole wheat or other whole grain bread,
and meat, with eggs twice a week, get every mineral salt needed by the body and every essential
vitamin. If they further take the precaution of eating salt-water fish—fish from the ocean—once or
twice a week, they make assurance doubly sure."

We might add that baked or broiled liver once
a week is added insurance, for the liver is the great
chemical factory of the body and full of vital compounds.

ADVICE ON SUPPLEMENTARY VITAMINS AND MINERALS

But what of those who feel they must "take something" because they have remedies so strongly in mind? Our habit has been and still is to tell them to take one dose of Multivitamins a day; every large maker of vitamins makes up some kind of Multi-vitamin preparation, containing all vitamins that have so far been proved essential to human welfare. Take an ordinary dose of this daily, but do not make the mistake of taking what is called massive dosage, going into more than 100,000 units daily. Many who sell foods advise this, but it is a bad thing to do—keep to the ordinary dosage unless a real doctor tells you to take more, and if he gives you many thousand units daily, ask him how long you are to keep up the large dosage. There should always be a termination to heavy dosage. The average dose will not harm, as the heavy dosage can and does.

Another simple remedy may be brewer's yeast, a few tablets per day. This is very rich in vitamins, especially those in the B group.

And then there are those who fear they will be short of minerals. We often tell them to get powdered kelp, and either take a moderate amount of it daily with water or juice, or use it as seasoning in place of table salt. In the work of helping human beings to better health it is as necessary to satisfy the mind as it is to direct them to improved physical health.

No matter how this book is arranged, this is the chapter that is written last. So we wish to remind you once more of a great truth: Human beings have a strong tendency to go to extremes, and to narrow down the truth until it is not the truth any more. In natural living, or Nature's Way of dealing with disease, the human mind tends to leap to the conclusion that it is "all in the eating, all in food."

NOT ALL IN THE EATING

So please let us tell you what we have surely told you before: Health is as broad as life itself. So we have to take all the factors into consideration, the physical, the mental-emotional, and even the spiritual ones. Some years ago we had grounded an insurance agent in such truth and had helped to bring him back to health, using much psychology in so doing. On his last professional visit we made a broad summary of the truth about health, and the patient replied with a broad grin, "That is right, doctor; it is all in the eating, isn't it?"

Our answer was, "No, it is not; it is partly in the eating, but it is also in the breathing, and exercising, and eliminating so as to have internal cleanliness, and in the drinking; it is also in the emotional and thought direction, so the mind works in constructive, health-building ways most of the time. And with some it is in the direction of the spiritual life. The chief cause of your illness was the depression, worry, fear and anxiety that ruled your life, and made your body sick. Have you already forgotten our hardest and most important work with you, helping to get your mind away from the depressive, destructive side of life and into the positive way of emotional and thought expression? No, it is not all in the eating."

And another great difficulty we have had with thousands of arthritics—they would read our instructions and continue to live in the bad old way that made them sick.

There is health in these pages, but merely reading them will help you not one iota. You have to live the teachings in these pages to obtain results. And you have to persist and persevere in right, natural living to obtain and maintain health.

III FOODS AND COOKING

17 Foods and Cooking

PROTEINS

The principal sources of protein are:

1 Meats of all kinds (the lean part), such as beef, veal, mutton, lean pork, chicken, turkey, duck, goose, game, both feathered and furred, in fact, all lean flesh from animals and birds.

2 Fish of all kinds, such as trout, salmon, herring, pickerel, pike, cod, halibut, mackerel, sturgeon, and shad. Also shellfish, like oysters (which are mostly water), clams, crabs and lobsters.

3 Legumes, the chief of which are dried beans, dried peas, lentils and peanuts. Also green peas, and both the green and the dried lima beans. Soybeans are included.

4 Dairy products, including sweet milk, clabbered milk, buttermilk, yogurt, cottage cheese

and all other kinds of cheese. Cream contains
but little protein, and butter practicaly none.
5 Nuts, especially almonds, Brazil nuts, filberts,
hickory nuts, pecans, English walnuts, butternuts, pistachios and pignolias. However, most
nuts are richer in oil than in protein.

STARCHES

The chief sources of our starchy foods are:
1 Cereals, the most important being wheat, In-
dian corn, rice, rye, barley, oats. No matter in
what form we eat them—in bread, cakes, mushes, flaked or puffed cereals—they are starchy.
2 Tubers, the most important being white potatoes, sweet potatoes and yams.
3 Legumes, especially the dried ones. The ripe
limas, navy beans and other kinds of ripe beans,
peas, lentils, soybeans and peanuts are starchy.
Green limas and young peas contain more
starch than the other vegetables usually classified as succulent.
4 Nuts, but only a few varieties. Acorns, dried
chestnuts and coconuts are rich in starch.
Green bananas are about as starchy as white
potatoes, but ripe bananas contain only a trace
of starch, for it has been turned to sugar.
Parsnips are rich in starch.

Pumpkins are of watery consistency, and may be classed with the succulent vegetables.

Tapioca and sago are very starchy.

Corn starch is the starchy essence of the corn.

Spaghetti and macaroni are cereals, hence starchy.

SUGARS

The principal sources of sugars are:

1 Sweet fruits, the most important of which are ripe bananas, currants, sweet grapes, raisins, sweet prunes, figs, dates and persimmons.

   All ripe fruits contain some sugar and the dried fruits are rich in this food element.

2 Sugar cane and sugar beets, from which nearly all of the refined white sugar is made.

3 Honey.

4 Sap of the sugar maple. Molasses.

FATS AND OILS

The chief sources of our fats are:

1 Dairy products—cream, butter and some rich cheeses.

2 Flesh of animals, especially pork, mutton and beef, that have been fattened.

3 Fat fish, such as herring, shad, salmon trout, tuna and salmon.

4 Legumes. Some peanuts are very oily, and so are soybeans.

5 Nuts of nearly every kind. Almonds, Brazil nuts, filberts, hickory nuts, pecans, English walnuts, butternuts, coconuts, and pistachios are rich in oil.

SUCCULENT VEGETABLES

The principal succulent vegetables are:

Asparagus, beets, cabbage, carrots, turnips, parsnips, cauliflower, cucumber, eggplant, lettuce, okra (gumbo), onions, radish, summer squash, tomatoes, spinach, kohlrabi, kale, Brussels sprouts, cone artichoke, chard, string beans, celery, turnip tops, lotus, endive, dandelion, oyster plant, rutabaga and garlic. Though corn is really a cereal, corn in the milk, either on the cob or canned, and green peas may also be classed with the succulent vegetables. Also the pumpkin.

Mushroom is a fungus. Those who are fond of it may partake, but fungus growths cannot be recommended as a steady diet.

Young lima beans are quite starchy. Parsnips are also rich in starch.

Radishes are delicious peeled and cooked.

Macaroni and spaghetti are *not* vegetables. They

are made of wheat and are very starchy. They are cereal food. So is rice.

RAW SALAD VEGETABLES

These are also succulent vegetables.

The principal salad vegetables are:

Lettuce, endive, romaine, chicory, tomatoes, cucumbers, cabbage, celery cabbage, parsley, field lettuce, cress. All leaves that are relished may be used for salad purposes.

Raw onions in moderation may be used for flavoring, and garlic likewise. Those who are fond of raw root vegetables and have good digestive power may eat raw carrots or turnips, but they should masticate these foods very well. Grated carrot tastes well in salads.

FRUITS

The term "acid fruit" means fruit that is quite sour, like sour apples, pineapples and lemons.

"Subacid fruit" is a mild fruit, containing only a little acid, such as mild pears, sweet apples and good blueberries.

Some of the most common *juicy fruits* are:

Apples, lemons, oranges, peaches, pears, strawberries, apricots, blackberries, cherries, cranber-

ries, currants, gooseberries, grapes, huckleberries,
blueberries, mulberries, nectarines, olives, pineapples, plums, raspberries and whortleberries.

The melons (watermelon, muskmelon, cantaloupe, casaba, honey dew, etc.), and tomatoes are
so like fruit that for practical purposes we may
call them so.

The most important *sweet fruits* are:

Ripe bananas, sweet prunes, sweet grapes, raisins, dried currants, figs, dates and persimmons.

COOKING HINTS

Just pause and consider a little. The human body is
composed of air, water and food. Food is the basis
of the material part of life. It is the stone and brick
and wood and glass and mortar and steel that enter into the building of our bodies. You have
watched builders erect various edifices. They do
not scramble their materials into a haphazard heap.
They know how and where to place the different
materials they use. They do not throw window
panes in the mortar; they do not attempt to attach
steel beams to each other by means of wooden
pegs; they do not scatter great blocks of stone on
the roof.

The human body is far more delicate, complex
and important than any edifice erected by man.

If you value this human structure of yours, supply to it the right kind of food, in correct combinations, in proper quantities, at propitious times. For some thousands of years a few individuals have known that right feeding is the most important factor in maintaining physical health, or in regaining lost health. So we are giving you these pointers on food preparation.

MEAT: Prepare by stewing, baking in the oven, roasting in the old fashion before or above an open fire, broiling or steaming. Or use a fireless cooker or a pressure cooker. If you use either of the latter two methods you will find directions accompanying the utensils, but you need not season as they direct. The proper way to obtain a tender, juicy piece of meat its to apply high heat in the very beginning, for about fifteen minutes in case it is a moderate sized piece of meat, and then finish the cooking at a low temperature. If you place a piece of meat in a cool oven, gradually raise the temperature and finish with high heat, you are apt to have a tough, dry roast. If you put the meat into a piping hot oven the heat sears the surface and keeps the juices in the meat.

Season in moderation always.

To mix greasy meat juices with flour and other starches, making thickened gravy, or brown gravy, is a mistake from the standpoint of health. Cooking grease into flour or into other starch, produces food that builds arthritis and other ills.

Frying is the most objectionable mode of cooking. The process of frying renders a part of the food indigestible, and after a while helps to ruin the digestive apparatus. "But I do not fry in lard; I use butter," some say, thinking this makes the process all right. It is not the source of the fat that is objectionable, it is the frying process itself. Butter-fried foods are as bad as lard-fried ones. Others are still more virtuous and say: "I don't use animal grease; I fry in olive oil." Again, it is not the source of the fat that is objectionable; it is the frying process itself that is bad. Don't fry anything if you are desirous of building the best of health. Avoid greasy cooking.

Season the meats when the cooking process is almost finished, or let each individual do most of the seasoning at the table. Pepper, mustard, sharp sauces and hot condiments are irritants which overstimulate the appetite, lead to overeating and hurt the digestive organs.

Pickled and preserved meats are rather poor foods, and should seldom be used.

Arthritic subjects should not eat meat more than once a day.

FISH is best boiled, steamed, broiled or baked. Fish easily becomes tainted, so select it with care to see that it is fresh.

EGGS may be prepared in your favorite way, with the exception that they are not to be cooked in grease. Greasing the pan enough to keep the eggs (or other foods) from sticking does no harm. Eggs may be made into omelettes or scrambled. But to cook eggs in sputtering grease is wrong.

Soft boiled eggs, poached eggs and coddled eggs are easy to digest.

If properly prepared, hard boiled eggs are also easy to digest. The wrong way to cook a hard boiled egg is to leave it in boiling water five or six minutes. The right way is to cook it slowly twenty minutes. Then it becomes mealy and tender.

POTATOES are best baked, or boiled in the jacket or steamed. If potatoes are peeled, soaked in cold water and then cooked, they lose a large part of their nutritive value and a very large portion of their health-bearing virtues—natural salts and vitamins.

If potatoes are well scrubbed and baked, they may be eaten peeling and all. From the standpoint of health, the best portion of the potato is close to the skin. No fried potatoes.

BREAD should be made as near as possible from whole grain flour, that is, flour made by grinding the entire grain. White flour products are very easy to digest but they are poor foods. Refined flour is poor in mineral elements, poor in the vitamins that build rich blood and strength and health. It is a blood-starving food.

Whole wheat flour products are a little harder to digest than the white flour foods, but ordinary digestion takes care of the whole grain products, and they build health.

Yeast bread should be stale before it is consumed, and always well masticated.

Toasting starts the digestive process by changing a part of the bread starch into a form of sugar. The best method of toasting is to slice stale bread fairly thin and put it into a slow oven until it is crisped throughout.

MUFFINS, GEMS, BAKING POWDER BISCUITS AND SODA BISCUITS may be safely eaten fresh, provided they are made thin, well baked and thoroughly masticated. They take the place of bread.

CORN BREAD should be made thin and baked crisp and crusty. It should be extra well masticated.

To use sugar, jelly, jam and fruit preserves on bread is a mistake, for it results in abnormal fermentation and production of an excessive amount of acid and gas in the digestive organs. This helps to build catarrh in those who have a catarrhal tendency.

COOKED CEREALS, that is, mushes made of whole grains, such as oats or whole wheat, are good food provided no sugar is added to them, and further provided that they are thoroughly masticated. It should require fifteen minutes to eat a dish of such cooked cereal. Cereal mushes are starchy and should be well mixed with saliva. Otherwise they readily go into abnormal fermentation. Take no bread or toast in the meal, if you eat a breakfast cereal.

WHITE OR REFINED SUGAR is one of our health problems. A person quickly acquires a taste for sugar. It quickly digests, and can in a short time be turned into heat and energy.

Its great fault is that it is almost a pure carbon, a dead food, devoid of all health-giving properties. From the health standpoint it is the worst of all our staples. We ought to obtain our sugar from berries, melons and fruits; also from honey, maple sugar and the dark sugars. Instead of eating a hundred pounds of white sugar apiece each year, as Americans do, we should eat natural sweets.

VEGETABLES: The basic recipe for vegetable cooking is to clean, cut if necessary, and cook in so little water that there is none to drain off after cooking, adding nothing except salt to taste; when the vegetables are done, add such dressing as butter or oil, or other desired fat. Eat your share of the cooking liquor.

Cover the pot in which the vegetables are

cooked, for open pot cooking results in the oxidizing of many vitamins.

Cook in covered pot, or steam or bake, or in fireless cooker or pressure cooker. The pressure cooker preserves the vital elements in vegetables better than other methods, for the oxygen is largely exhausted before the cooking begins. It is not so much the heat as the oxidation that destroys the vitamins. Overcooking is undesirable. The frozen vegetables are excellent. Do not prethaw them. Always take your share of the cooking liquor, for it contains much of the natural mineral salts and vitamins.

Cooked vegetables and raw salad vegetables should make up the larger part of both the lunch and the dinner, for these foods are so helpful in building good blood and wholesome body, also in normalizing the bowels, that they are invaluable in regaining lost health, or in maintaining what health one has.

Greens, like spinach, chard, tender beet tops, tender turnip tops and young kale, should be cooked only a short time—some of these tender leafy greens need only from three to five minutes of cooking. They need almost no water in the pot to cook, for they are so full of juice. The leafy greens are especially valuable, for they are rich in calcium and other mineral salts—so many persons are afraid of being short of calcium—the leafy greens, the raw salad vegetable and fruits and whole wheat bread are some solutions to allay this fear.

VITAMINS: These are complex chemicals present in our foods. For instance, Vitamin A is abundant in the green and yellow vegetables; the B Complex is found in such foods as liver, eggs, peanuts and yeast; Vitamin C is abundant in tomatoes, oranges and other fruits; Vitamin D is present in butter and other fatty foods—it is also created by sunshine acting on the ergosterol in the skin; Vitamin E is so abundant in many foods that we can forget about it; it is plentiful in wheat germ, which we get in whole wheat bread.

The point is that vitamins are abundantly present in natural foods, but they are either absent or too greatly diminished in some of the highly processed foods. White sugar contains no vitamins, no organic mineral salts; in white flour many of the precious vitamins and organic mineral salts, essential to health building, have vanished; the precious wheat germ is absent in white flour. This is the reason we recommend the eating of natural foods. They furnish the vital compounds that are needed to build and maintain health.

This is also the reason we recommend simple cooking, and the eating of raw fruits and raw vegetable salads, for in this way the body obtains the compounds needed to overcome arthritis and other ills.

To bring this subject down to earth: Eat fruits daily, at least one good serving being raw; have raw vegetable salad once or twice daily; have cooked vegetables twice a day; avoid white bread and take the whole wheat bread instead; have the potatoes baked or cooked in the jacket; do your cooking as recommended in this book; avoid cake, cookies, pies and puddings, and use fruits, including melons and berries, as your dessert. Do this, and you will get all the vitamins you need, and supply the body's essential mineral salts, also chlorophyll.

This is not saying that vitamins in moderation do not help some sick persons. But whatever you do, avoid the massive doses of vitamins recommended to you by laymen. At present I have a patient who was made very ill by massive doses of Vitamin D—they poisoned her. In ordinary dosage, vitamins have no toxic effects.

Eat right, and you get your vitamins and mineral salts in the normal way, that is, in your foods. If you live in a goitre belt, use iodized salt so as to obtain the normal amount of iodine.

VEGETABLE SALADS: For a list of these vegetables see the paragraphs under the heading of Raw Salad Vegetables.

The raw vegetables contain salts and juices that help to keep the body alkaline and pure and healthy. Raw vegetables should form a part of at least one meal daily. It would be fine to serve them twice a day. They are rich in vitamins.

Some find it trying to digest raw cabbage and raw onions. But the average digestive apparatus will take good care of lettuce, celery and other leafy salad vegetables. The raw leafy vegetables that the individual relishes and is able to digest make good salad materials. Those who have excellent digestion may add raw root vegetables to their salad, such as carrots, turnips and radishes; or cucumbers; or any other raw vegetable that pleases the taste. Raw vegetables should be well masticated.

It is best to eat only two to four vegetables in a salad, but if the digestion is good, there may be greater variety.

The chief reason for eating raw vegetables is to furnish elements to keep the blood in its normal alkaline reaction, and vital. Those who want to make their foods sour should use lemon juice, or grapefruit juice, or pineapple juice, or the juice of any other tart fruit. Fruit acids do not acidulate the body. Those who like mixed salad dressings should know that lemon juice may be employed where vinegar has been used in the past. Many enjoy raw vegetables without dressing. A little salt may be used; or salt and oil; or salt, oil and lemon juice, or lemon juice and salt.

The greatest blood-purifying aid is obtained when the salad ingredients are raw. Then they are richer in vitamins.

Fruit salads are best when the fruits or berries used are raw. A liberal amount of lettuce or celery mixed with the fruit improves the salad as a health-builder.

FRUITS: They are best raw, without sugar. Much fruit is spoiled by being made into jelly, jam and preserves. Canned vegetables are quite good when fresh ones are out of the question, but canned fruits often ferment too easily in the digestive tract. If fresh fruits are not to be had, get a supply of good dried fruits, or evaporated fruits. Unfortunately, most of the frozen fruits are put up in white sugar.

Fruits are health builders when they are not ruined in preparation and combination. The chief mistake is to dose them with white sugar. Raisins, figs and dates may be used as sweeteners. In baking apples, for instance: Core the apples, and fill the centers with well soaked raisins, using the juice for dressing or sauce on the apple. (If the raisins are not soaked they will not sweeten the apple.) The results are good.

The fresh fruits and vegetables help to purify the blood and the whole body. They are rich in the essential organic mineral salts and vitamins, especially the leafy vegetables. They are health builders.

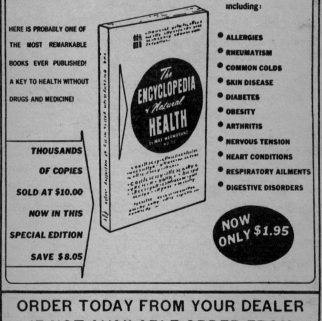